Foods
That
Cause
You to
Lose
Weight

The Negative Calorie Effect

Neal D. Barnard, M.D.

Design by Mercedes Everett

Printed in the U.S.A.
ISBN 1-882330-35-8
Second Edition

CONTENTS

PREFACE

The popularity of <u>Foods That Cause You to Lose Weight</u>, with more than a million copies in print, is due to the fact that it is very effective and remarkably easy. Thanks to research at major medical centers which you will read about in this volume, we now have a much better understanding of what causes weight problems and how to conquer them. Getting lasting results is so much easier than struggling with old-fashioned diets, a wonderful relief if you have been through the diet routine a time or two.

The outcome of this research is a breakthrough called the negative calorie effect. It does not mean that some foods have no calories. It means that certain foods are naturally modest in calories and that they actually increase your calorie-burning speed for hours after a meal. Moreover, certain nutrients tend not to add to your body fat. If your body were to try to make fat out of them, just the process of building fat molecules consumes a substantial number of their calories.

The negative calorie effect allows you to lose weight without counting calories or setting strict limits on how much you eat, and lets you enjoy eating again.

This program is completely different from others. You may find it surprising, and it will certainly lead you to a very different way of thinking about foods. Let me encourage you to read over the basic concepts in this book so you understand how it works. Then just try it for three weeks. Think of this program as an experiment. If you try it very carefully for just three weeks, you will very likely wish you had tried it long ago.

This new edition has been completely revised and expanded. The menus and recipes have been thoroughly revamped with an eye toward ease of preparation, maximizing the negative calorie effect, and delighting the taste buds with a minimum of preparation time.

I hope you will let me know how things go for you. You can write to me at Box 6322, Department A, Washington, D.C. 20015. I regret to say that sometimes the deluge of mail I receive makes it difficult to respond personally, but I do look forward to hearing from you, because your experience helps refine this program for other people.

I owe a debt of gratitude to Evan Reynolds, Bob and Cynthia Holzapfel, and Richard Muldawer, without whose support and expertise this volume would never have been possible. Particular appreciation also goes to the many researchers who laid the groundwork for the medical breakthrough that has put permanent weight control within reach as never before, and whose published works are listed in the reference section. Special thanks to Jennifer Raymond, whose unparalleled culinary wisdom and experience translated these medical principles into menus and recipes that are easy to make and every bit as delightful as they are powerful.

Neal D. Barnard, M.D.

NOTICE TO THE READER

Learning to tap the power of foods can be enormously rewarding. Even so, neither this book nor any other can substitute for individual medical attention and advice. If you have any medical condition, are significantly overweight, or are on medication, you should consult your doctor as you plan changes in your diet. Dietary changes can sometimes change your need for medication or have other important effects. You should also see your doctor before any substantial increase in your physical activity if you are over forty or have any medical condition.

If you are pregnant or nursing, or if you follow this program strictly for more than three years, please consult the information on vitamin B_{12} on page 58.

INTRODUCTION

This book offers a new approach to weight control. If your goal is a slimmer body and more energy than you have had in years, this program is more powerful than any diet you have ever tried. In fact, it is not a "diet." It is a nutritional breakthrough that brings about better weight control than old-fashioned diets ever could.

This book was written because typical diets have not been very successful. Many are simply too weak to get results. Others use an artificial formula approach that no one could live with permanently. They may cause weight loss for a few weeks, often followed by weight gain back to and beyond the starting point. This frustrating result is caused by the poor design of the diets.

This book is based on a revolution in our understanding of how foods affect our weight. Researchers have tested many different kinds of diets: diets to help people lower their blood pressure or cholesterol levels, or deal with various other health problems. In the course of these studies, people eating certain kinds of foods started losing weight--sometimes phenomenal amounts of weight. They were not counting calories or limiting the size of their meals, yet the pounds came off. The weight loss was caused, not by restricting the amount of food they ate, which is the usual approach, but by changing the type of food they ate. It turns out that certain foods cannot add directly or easily to body fat. Even better, they actually increase your metabolism so that you burn calories faster for hours after the meal.

One important example comes from researchers with the National Institutes of Health, who found that when certain types of food make up the daily menu, people lose weight even when they do not put any limit on how much they eat.[1]

Similarly, Dean Ornish, M.D., a well-known researcher on the faculty of the University of California at San Francisco, has shown how weight loss can result, sometimes quite dramatically, even when people eat more than they were eating previously. Dr. Ornish used a specially designed set of dietary guidelines to help patients with heart disease. Although he encouraged his patients to pay attention to the type of food they ate, there was no limit on how much they could eat. They could eat until they were full and never had to count calories, skip meals, shy away from having seconds, or endure any of the other punishments that are common on old-fashioned diets.

The results were astounding. Not only did their heart health improve dramatically; they also started losing weight. Of course, those who were already at a healthy weight did not lose more weight. But those who had a few pounds to lose--or more than a few--started losing weight automatically. After the first year, one patient had lost nearly 100 pounds, and the average patient had lost 22 pounds without dieting in the old sense of the term.[2]

You do not have to be involved in a research study to get results that can be breath-taking. Take Leslie, for example. She had been up and down the scale dozens of times, struggling to lose weight, only to find the weight return sooner or later. Like most people in this situation, she felt more and more discouraged. Several of her relatives had weight problems that led to heart disease and other deadly health concerns, and she feared that the same fate was in store for her.

Then she learned the principles you will read about shortly. She focused on adjusting the type of food she ate and, in the process, gained a dramatically new level of control over her weight. She lost 94 pounds, and did so without ever counting a calorie. In the pictures she sent me, she was certainly slimmer. Her chin was nicely tucked in, and her waistline had slimmed dramatically. But her pictures also showed a look of confidence that comes from finally learning the secrets of conquering weight problems.

One very important point: You do not have to decide to change the way you eat forever. All I ask you to do is to try this program for three weeks. For just 21 days, give it a good test. If you like the results, stick with it. But there is no need to make any long-term commitments now. Just give it a try. This program brings you the negative calorie effect in an easy, step-by-step method. First, we will clear away the myths that have led people to punish themselves with diets that work poorly, if at all, and often do more harm that good. Then, we will look at how to use the elegantly simple, but powerful, negative calorie effect. If compulsive eating is your problem, we will review the two-pronged approach that has helped so many people break out of that trap. You'll have plenty of quick, delicious, and healthful menus and recipes that use the negative calorie effect and make eating a joy. We will also add a simple, optional program for physical activity for those who want to maximize their gains.

When you put this program to work, you can have the slimmest body nature ever intended for you. Get all you can out of it. No corners were cut in bringing this information to you, and you will not want to cut any corners in putting it into action.

You can succeed. So be patient, and do not rush. It took time for you to gain weight, and it will take time for it to come off again. Let the pounds come off gradually, but surely. I think you will be happy with the new you.

Foods That Cause You to Lose Weight

1

CLEAR AWAY THE DIET MYTH

Your body is always changing. Like a sculptor perfecting a work in progress, adding a bit of clay here and paring some away there, your body works with its own raw materials--oxygen, water, and foods--to continually remodel your bones, muscles, fat layer, and skin. Just as the right materials make the artist's job easy, the same is true for your body. Certain foods help you sculpt your body, so to speak, while other foods make the job difficult, or even impossible.

In this book, we will cover the factors that affect your weight to a surprising degree. But first, we need to clear away a few myths. Most people try to carve away unwanted pounds by going on diets. Small portions of food and persistent hunger are tolerated in the hope that, if not much food is coming in, fat will have to be burned.

Personal experience and a wealth of scientific study show that diets are about as useful for weight control as a wrecking ball is for classical sculpture. Let's take a minute to understand why diets present such difficulties. Then we will look in detail at what really does work.

If you have ever been on a diet, did you find the results to be something other than lasting success? If so, you may find it re-assuring to know that the problem was not weak will power or poor self-discipline. The problem was the diet itself.

The human body took shape millions of years ago, long before diets were invented. At that time, the lack of food meant only one thing: starvation. If the body could not cope with the lack of food, the result was life-threatening. So we have built-in mechanisms to preserve ourselves in times of shortages. These defenses automatically go to work any time your food intake is low. When you go on a low-calorie diet, you know that you are trying to lose weight. But your body does not know that. As far as your body is concerned, you are starving, and it automatically tries to preserve the very fat you are trying to get rid of. To do that, it does something you definitely do not want. It burns calories slower.

The speed at which your body burns calories is called your metabolic rate. It is like the rate at which an automobile uses up gas. An idling car uses up some fuel. When the car is moving it uses more, and when it accelerates up a hill it will use a lot more. Our bodies work the same way. We burn some calories even when we are relaxing or asleep because it takes energy to maintain our body temperature and to keep our lungs, heart, brain and other organs working. When we get up and move around, we burn more calories. The more we move, the more calories we burn.

Some people have a "fast metabolism" and burn lots of calories in a short time. They are likely to stay slim. Other people have a slower metabolism and have a harder time staying slim. But in either case, your metabolism can change. For many people, it slows as they get older. In this book, you will learn how your metabolism can actually speed up to help you burn fat.

DIETS SLOW YOUR METABOLISM

Remember the last time you were driving along and suddenly noticed that the gas gauge was below empty? You went easy on the accelerator, driving very smoothly, and turned off the engine at stop lights to conserve gas until you got to a station. Your body does the same thing when you diet. It recognizes that food is in short supply, so it turns down your metabolism to save as much of your fat as possible until normal eating returns. Fat is your fuel reserve, and while you are trying hard to get rid of it, your body is doing everything it can to hold on to it. It is trying to save you from starvation.

A research team at the University of California at Los Angeles put a group of young women on an 800-calorie-per-day diet for three weeks. They found that their calorie-burning speed fell by 13 percent, on average. They then asked these women to exercise to see if that would counteract the slowed metabolism. It did not. The body fights diets so hard that it will keep the metabolism slow to save body fat, even in the face of vigorous exercise.[3]

This can be very frustrating. Dieters often find that, even though they eat very little, their bodies do not easily shed the pounds. Even worse, the slowed metabolism continues beyond the dieting period, often for weeks, according to studies at the University of Pennsylvania and elsewhere.[4] So weight easily returns after a diet. This causes the familiar "yo-yo" phenomenon, in which dieters lose some weight, then rebound to a higher weight than they started with.

Let's look at how this works by visiting the home of a fictitious couple whom we'll call Bill and Susan. Bill has gained a bit of weight over the last several years, so he decided to try a program that consisted of diet milkshakes. "One for breakfast, another for lunch, followed by a sensible dinner," the instructions said. Even with the optional diet "candy bar" that he was allowed in the afternoon, it was a tedious routine. He had a smoldering hunger all day long, and a "sensible" dinner did not seem to be enough after a day of near-starvation. He started to feel out of sorts and a bit cranky. He might also have become a bit constipated, because Susan noticed that he had moved a magazine rack into the bathroom.

But Bill really tried to stick with it. In fact, Susan could swear she once woke up to hear him mumbling in his sleep, "One for breakfast, another for lunch, and a sensible dinner. One for breakfast, another for lunch, and a sensible dinner."

Bill did lose a few pounds at first. But as time went on, his weight seemed to get stuck. It just would not drop any lower. After a couple of weeks, he quit the diet and went back to his normal way of eating. Not surprisingly, his weight drifted back up to where it had been. But what he had not counted on was that his weight kept increasing <u>beyond</u> his starting weight. It was as if the diet had actually harmed his body's ability to burn calories, which is exactly what it had done. Susan still hears him cursing whenever he stands on the bathroom scale.

As Bill learned the hard way, the first step is to keep your calorie-burning speed up by keeping your body's anti-starvation mechanisms turned off. Here is how to do it: Make sure that your daily diet contains at least 10 calories per pound of your ideal body weight. This means that if you are aiming for a weight of 150 pounds, your daily menu should contain at least 1,500 calories. If you are aiming for a weight of 120 pounds, your diet should have 1,200 calories or more. This is a minimum. There is no set maximum, as we will see shortly. That way, you will not slow your metabolism, and you will be able to retain your progress. If you eat less than the 10-calories-per-pound guideline, your metabolism is likely to slow down.

DIETS LEAD TO BINGES

There is another problem with skimpy eating. Not only does your body slow down your calorie burning to hang on to body fat; it also encourages you to binge, in what is called the "restrained-eater" phenomenon. Bill learned about this, too. After he had been on the diet for several days and was good and hungry, Susan made the mistake of bringing home a carton of ice cream.

Unbeknownst to Bill, his body had been on the lookout for food, like a starving person trudging through a desert--primed and ready to gorge on whatever came his way. This is the body's second anti-starvation defense. If food is so rare that your body senses the risk of starvation, your hunger drive is automatically reset to make you likely to binge on any food you find.

A little bit won't hurt, Bill figured, as he opened the ice cream carton and dug the spoon in. But before he knew it, he had eaten his serving and part of Susan's, and was digging the spoon back into the carton. Soon, he was running the spoon around the cracks in the bottom, trying to get every last bit. He tore the carton apart and licked the sides.

He then felt terribly guilty, and scolded himself for his lack of will power. But the real problem was not will power at all. The "problem" was the innate biological programming of the human body. The diet turned on the normal anti-starvation defenses that were built into his body, as they are in every human being. His body assumed that he was starving and this might be the only food he would find for a while, so it demanded a binge. The same thing can happen if you skip meals. Skipping breakfast or lunch leads to overeating later in the day.

Sometimes binging gets really out of control. Bulimia-- binge-eating often followed by purging--almost always begins with a diet. And when binging begins, shame and secrecy often follow. If this has happened to you, remember that binging is not a moral failing. It is a natural consequence of dieting.

The cultural trend in Western countries in the past several decades has emphasized meat, dairy products, fried foods, and other high-fat foods. Combined with an increasingly sedentary lifestyle, the predictable result is that many people become overweight. They mistakenly believe that the problem is the amount of food they are eating, rather than the type of food. Rather than abandon the offending foods, they simply eat smaller amounts. The natural result is lowered metabolism, cravings, binges, and failure. The more we diet, the more we slow our natural calorie-burning ability, and the more likely we are to binge.

Happily, skipping meals and eating minuscule portions are completely unnecessary. As we will see, there is a much better way.

2

HOW TO USE THE NEGATIVE
CALORIE EFFECT

Now that you know what not to do, let's build a program that takes pounds off and helps you keep them off. The first step is to look at what foods are made of, and how these nutrients affect your ability to burn calories and, ultimately, your weight. We'll keep things simple, but I do want you to understand the logic behind this program.

Foods are mainly made up of four things: carbohydrate, protein, fat, and water, along with much smaller amounts of vitamins, minerals, and fiber. Dietitians keep charts showing exactly how much of each of these nutrients is in thousands of different foods, because they know that different nutrients have dramatically different effects on the body.

Carbohydrate, for example, is the fuel that keeps your body running. The white inside of a potato is mostly complex carbohydrate, which you might also call starch. Rice, breads, pasta, beans, and most vegetables are rich in complex carbs. When you eat any of these foods, their carbohydrate is gradually broken apart and absorbed to provide energy.

Although your car can burn just about any kind of fuel, albeit with a bit of difficulty, it runs much smoother on the grade of gasoline it was designed for. Your body is the same way. You could survive--although not very well--by eating nothing but hot dogs and chicken wings, but the fuel your body burns easily and efficiently comes from carbohydrates.

Proteins are very different. They are like spare parts, providing the structural material to build and repair your body. Protein's microscopic strands are found in virtually all foods. While many people think of protein as coming from meats or eggs, it is also in all vegetables, grains, fruits, and beans. It is what makes a carrot's shape different from a radish.

Fat is like the oil and lubrication of your car. You need a little of it for things to run smoothly, but a little bit goes a very long way. If it is dripping all over the place, it causes problems.

The most valuable foods for people who want to lose weight are those rich in carbohydrates. These starchy potatoes, rice, pasta, beans, and vegetables seem humble. But to your body they are like the finest slimming formula in the world. Complex carbs have a feature that you will not find in any other nutrient. Your body can use the energy they provide and easily keep them from adding to your body fat.

In the past, many people believed that potatoes, rice, bread, and pasta were fattening. But the fact is, carbohydrates are very modest in calories. A baked potato has less than 100 calories. A piece of bread has 70 calories. A half-cup of rice has only about 110.

Compare them with fats or oils. While one gram (1/28 ounce) of carbohydrate has only four calories, a gram of fat or oil has nine. And while a half-cup of rice has only 110 calories, a half-cup of chicken fat or corn oil has, believe it or not, 960 calories. To put it another way, there are more calories in just one tablespoon of any fat or oil than are in a whole potato, a slice of bread, or a half-cup of pasta. As we will see, many foods contain surprising amounts of fat that, over the long run, can spell weight problems.

Researchers with the National Institutes of Health found that when carbohydrate-rich foods are added to the diet in place of fatty foods, people lose weight, even when they are not consciously limiting how much they eat.[1] As we will see, even if you occasionally keep eating high-carb foods well past the point when you are full, your body will not turn the carbohydrate to fat.[5]

Complex carbs are plentiful in most foods from plants, but are never found in animal products. Fish, chicken, beef, and eggs are mainly protein and fat. That is why a chicken breast, which contains no carbohydrate, has fully 386 calories. If, instead, there were complex carbs in chicken, its calorie content would be much lower. But no animal product contains complex carbs.

CARBOHYDRATES CANNOT ADD DIRECTLY TO FAT

Carbohydrates cannot add easily to your body fat. You do not have any "carbohydrate storage areas" on your waistline or thighs. Let's say that, as an experiment, you were to eat a huge amount of spaghetti, curried rice, or potatoes. If you overdo it a bit, your body burns off the excess by stepping up its carbohydrate-burning speed. If you <u>really</u> overdo it, your body converts some of the carbs into <u>glycogen</u>, which are quick energy molecules, rather like spare batteries kept in your muscles and liver. You may have heard of marathon runners "carbo-loading"--intentionally increasing the amount of glycogen in their muscles and liver to improve their endurance. Your body does the same thing when it has extra carbohydrate on board.

If your body were to try to store excess carbs as fat, it would have to break the carbohydrate molecules apart and make fat molecules out of them. This is not so easy for your body to do. The process of breaking apart carbohydrates to make fat burns up to 25% of their calories.

The result of all these factors is clear: extra calories from carbohydrates are not nearly as likely to increase body fat as are the same number of calories from fats.[5,6]

A team of Swiss scientists fed high-carb foods to a group of research subjects far in excess of what they needed. They found that, indeed, the body responds by burning carbohydrate faster and also stores some of it as glycogen. Only when these compensatory mechanisms are exceeded does the body start to build fat from the excess carbohydrate, and even then, the process of making fat molecules uses up a fair number of its calories.[5] In reality, most of us never come close to that point.

This is news to many people. Dieters used to assume that if two foods had the same number of calories, they would be equally fattening. Not true. Complex carbs are not likely to be turned to fat. And if your body does try to make fat from them, up to a quarter of their calories are eliminated in the process.

People used to blame starchy foods for weight problems. But we now know that starches were actually innocent bystanders. People would take a baked potato, which has only 95 calories, and top it with butter, sour cream, grated cheese, or bacon bits. As they gained weight, they blamed the potato. But what was fattening was not the potato, but the butter or other greasy toppings that were added to it. The same thing happens when butter or other fats are added to bread, spaghetti, corn, or other high-carb foods. Without all that grease, high-carb foods are slimming foods.

Charlene: Beating a Weight Problem

Charlene was a secretary at a university in Washington, D.C. She wanted to lose 30 pounds and, in fact, had wanted to lose the same 30 pounds for several years. Although she was not nearly as overweight as some people she knew, she felt self-conscious. Her six-year-old son kept asking why she didn't like to go to the swimming pool; in fact, she had thrown away her swimsuit in a fit of annoyance a couple of years ago. She had tried many different diets, formula drinks, and diet pills. All had promised success, but none worked over the long run.

When I met her, she was trying an ultra-high-protein diet that she had read about in a magazine. She skipped breakfast, had yogurt and turkey slices for lunch, and usually ate frozen dietetic meals for dinner. Her weight had stayed essentially the same. I suggested that, instead, she make complex carbohydrates the center of her diet, and take some other steps you will read about shortly. Breakfast was to be hot cereal, such as oatmeal or Cream of Wheat with sliced bananas, along with toast, and melon or strawberries. At work, she could have instant soup, salad, and a bean burrito (without the cheese) from the taco shop next door. For dinner, she could have a salad, pasta, and garlic bread, or maybe veggie chili, rice pilaf, or potatoes, along with plenty of vegetables, with fruit for dessert. Because this "diet" included a rather large quantity of food, she worried that she might actually gain weight on it. But simple calculations showed that, properly prepared, the calorie content of this menu was actually very modest. She lost weight gradually, and before long the 30 extra pounds were gone. She's ready to buy a new swimsuit.

A Natural Metabolism Boost

That high-carb spaghetti, rice pilaf, bean chili, baked potato, or bread has another advantage. It actually boosts your metabolism, speeding up your calorie-burning for hours after a meal. Here is how it works: Carbohydrates increase your natural production of two hormones, called thyroid hormone and noradrenaline, both of which step-up your metabolism. The result is faster calorie burning that begins automatically. The increased metabolism peaks at about 30 to 90 minutes and continues for hours after the meal.

For people who like technical explanations, here is what happens. Your thyroid gland is at the base of your neck, under your Adam's apple. It releases into the blood a weak hormone, called T_4. The name refers to the fact that four iodine atoms are attached to it. Carbohydrate-rich foods turn T_4 into a much more powerful hormone by removing one of these iodine atoms. The resulting hormone, now called T_3, increases the calorie-burning speed in your cells, just as stepping on the gas pedal of your car increases the rate at which the car burns gas. So high-carb foods are great for calorie burning.

Diets that are very low in complex carbs can do the opposite, turning T_4 into an inactive hormone called reverse T_3, slowing down your metabolism and short-circuiting your chance for success.

The thyroid boost is only half the story of your improved calorie-burning. Carbohydrate-rich foods also increase your body's production of another hormone, called noradrenaline, a close relative of adrenaline, and it adds to your ability to burn calories.[9]

So carbohydrate-rich foods are the best friends of anyone trying to slim down. They are naturally low in calories, they cannot easily add to your body fat, and they help boost your metabolism for hours, so calories are burned off faster.

Now here is a critical point: Complex carbohydrates are found only in plants. Grains, such as bread, spaghetti, and rice are loaded with them. The same is true of beans and vegetables. But, as I mentioned above, animal products are a different story altogether. There are no complex carbs in chicken, fish, beef, pork, eggs, or dairy products. The more animal products you put on your plate, the more carbohydrate-rich vegetable foods you are pushing off it. Even worse, because chicken, fish and other animal products do not have any complex carbs, they can encourage the inactivation of thyroid hormone, and your metabolism can actually slow down as a result. That is one reason why the most powerful weight-control programs use vegetarian menus.

There is an added bonus to foods from plants. They are rich in fiber, which adds a hearty texture to foods but has virtually no calories. Fiber is what people used to call roughage, the part of plants that resists digestion in the small intestine. Its value was not appreciated until relatively recently, and so it is often removed by refining methods. The result is white bread instead of whole-grain breads, white rice instead of brown rice, and baked goods that are more densely packed with calories and less satisfying than they should be. Like complex carbs, fiber is not found in fish or chicken or other animal products. It is found only in plants.

THE NEGATIVE CALORIE EFFECT

Many people still believe that the number of calories in any given food tells you just how fattening it is likely to be. For example, a cup of rice has about 220 calories. Three slices of bologna also have 220 calories. So you might assume that these two foods have exactly the same effect on your waistline.

They don't. The very same number of calories coming from bologna and from rice have very different effects. The bologna tends to be fattening, as a general rule, while the rice does not.

Rice does provide calories to run the body's functions. And theoretically it is possible for unused calories from rice to be stored as fat. But it turns out that rice is much less fattening than the same number of calories from bologna, other meats, or other fatty foods. Rice--like other high-carb foods--naturally reduces the calories that can affect your weight.

You can think of this as a "negative calorie effect." One of the most exciting concepts in the science of weight control in many years is the fact that certain foods can actually assist in the loss of fat.

The negative calorie effect does not mean that foods have zero calories, or less than zero. It means that foods that are loaded with complex carbs help you slim down in three ways:

First, they are naturally modest in calories.

Second, they tend not to add to body fat. As we saw earlier, your body resists turning carbohydrate into fat, and if it should try to break it down to make fat, up to 25% percent of its calories are lost in the process. That means that, of the 220 calories in a cup of rice, about 50 calories are subtracted if your body tries to convert them to fat. Leaving grains whole, like rice, cereals, or corn, rather than grinding them into flour to make bread or pasta, may also cause them to release fewer calories.

Third, they increase your metabolism, so calories are burned more quickly.

Another part of the negative calorie effect of carbohydrates is that they are the part of the diet that turns off your hunger drive.[11] When your body senses that it has gotten the carbs it needs, it reduces your appetite. The natural sugar in fruits, called fructose, also has an appetite-reducing effect.

Which foods have the negative calorie effect? As you know by now, you will not get it from fish, chicken, steak, or eggs, because there is virtually no complex carbohydrate in any animal product. Complex carbohydrates are found only in plants. Grains, vegetables, and beans are loaded with them.

Although dieters often feel that they should stop eating before they are satisfied, there is no need to limit yourself in that way. Just as your body cues you automatically to tell you how much air to breathe and how much water to drink, your body also guides you on how much to eat. That cuing mechanism works wonderfully when your menu is rich in high-carb foods, and it pays to listen to it.

Just as you need to follow your hunger drive, it is also important to pay attention to your satiety signal--the feeling of fullness that tells you when you've had enough. This is your body's cue that it is time for you to do something other than eat. If you continue eating long after you feel full and keep this up day after day, you will gain weight no matter what foods you eat. Although occasional overeating on high-carb foods does not cause weight gain, researchers at the University of Colorado pushed a group of volunteers to eat one and a half times their normal intake at every meal for two weeks, and found that even high-carbohydrate foods can cause weight gain when you really push it.[6] Even though they are never the problem that high-fat foods are, it is always important to follow your body's signals. That means eating when you are hungry and stopping when you are full.

30 Foods You Can Eat in Virtually Unlimited Portions

Listed below are 30 foods that you should feel free to eat in very generous portions. Unless you are really stuffing yourself well past the point when you are full, you can eat as much of these as you want. As noted above, pay attention to your natural hunger and satiety cues.

In fact, there are many more than 30. Nearly all plant foods--grains, beans, vegetables, and fruits--have the negative calorie effect. The primary exceptions are olives, avocados, seeds, nuts, and nut products, which are high in fat. One important caveat: Enjoy the negative calorie foods without butter, margarine, or oily toppings--fats can easily neutralize their benefit. You may think you can't live without those greasy foods, but you'll soon see how easy it can be.

Apples	Corn	Oatmeal
Bananas	Cream of Wheat	Oranges
Baked Beans	Cucumbers	Pasta noodles
Black Beans	Grapefruit	Peas
Broccoli	Grapes	Pineapple
Cabbage	Green beans	Pinto beans
Carrots	Kidney beans	Potatoes
Cauliflower	Lentils	Rice
Celery	Lettuce (all varieties)	Spinach
Cherries	Melons	Tomatoes

CUTTING OUT FATS AND OILS

Now that you have added foods that help you burn calories faster, there is a second vital step in slimming down. For while complex carbs are the raw materials your body needs to sculpt a slimmer body, fats and oils can destroy your artistry. You may have the bone structure and well-formed muscle layer of a Michelangelo statue, but this perfect body is easily hidden as fats and oils in the foods you eat cause your fat layer to expand.

They are, by far, the most fattening part of any food, and paring them off your menu helps keep them off your body. As we noted earlier, all fats hold more than double the calories, compared to carbohydrates. This is true for chicken fat, beef fat, fish oil, vegetable oil, and any other kind. They are loaded with calories, and they do nothing at all to improve your calorie-burning ability.[12] In addition, researchers have found that fatty foods can increase the appetite, making people eat more even after they are full.[13]

There are various kinds of fat. The main categories that dietitians are concerned with are saturated fats, which are common in animal products, and unsaturated fats, which are common in vegetable oils. Saturated fats are much worse for your heart, but for weight control, we need to be concerned about all fats and oils. All hold the same number of calories: nine in every gram.

It is surprising how much fat ends up on our plates. About 35-40 percent of the calories most people in Western countries get every day come from fat. For a typical 2000-calorie menu, that is 700-800 calories every day from nothing but fats and oils. By cutting most of them out, you can cut out hundreds of calories. To put it another way, when all the foods you eat are really low in fat, you can eat larger portions than you could on a high-fat diet, without more calories.

Researchers at Cornell University recently published the results of a fascinating experiment. They put volunteers on different diets for several weeks. They found that those whose meals were very low in fat and high in carbohydrates lost weight steadily without limiting how much they ate. But those on high-fat diets could not effectively lose weight even if they ate skimpy portions.

Cutting your fat intake from 35-40 percent of your daily calories down to about 10-15 percent is an easy, but powerful, weight-reducing step. It works hand-in-hand with the negative calorie effect. If you are eating high-carb foods and keeping fats and oils to a minimum, you are on the right track for success. But if you mix in fatty or oily foods, you can easily neutralize the negative calorie effect. So you want high-carb foods, and you also want to keep fats to a minimum.

To go on a "search and destroy" mission for fat, be on the look-out for the two forms it comes in: animal fat and vegetable oil. Let's take a look at both.

Animal Fat

Animal fat was designed by nature for one main purpose: to store calories for animals. When you eat animal fat, you are eating all those concentrated, stored-up calories. It is not only on the outside of a cut of meat. Fat is marbled through the lean, too, like water that has soaked through a sponge. That is true for chicken and turkey, just as it is for beef or pork. If you are eating meat, you are actually swallowing someone else's fat, and it can put fat on you.

Let's make a return visit to Bill and Susan's house, where our friends are making spaghetti--or to be more precise, Bill is clowning around in a chef's hat while Susan is cooking spaghetti. She is also making some fresh vegetables and opening a bottle of wine. Many people think of pasta as fattening, but a one-cup serving of spaghetti topped with 1/2 cup of tomato sauce has only about 200 calories. After all, spaghetti is made from wheat, so it's loaded with complex carbs and is only 4 percent fat. But if Susan had taken Bill's bad advice to add ground beef to the sauce, look what would have happened: the spaghetti dinner would suddenly have 365 calories. The fat in ground beef holds a lot of concentrated calories.

Let's take another example: A half-cup serving of mashed potatoes has only 70 calories. But add a tablespoon of butter on top and what happens? That bit of butter adds fully 108 calories, for a total of 178. Fatty toppings are high in calories, but the carbohydrate-rich potatoes, spaghetti, bread, etc., are not.

Dr. T. Colin Campbell runs the China Health Study, a massive and ongoing research undertaking. Most Chinese populations eat enormous amounts of rice or noodle dishes and plenty of vegetables, but very little in the way of animal products. As a result, their meals are very low in fat and are loaded with complex carbs. Dr. Campbell's research team found that, even though Chinese people eat more food, on average, than Westerners do, they stay much slimmer. That is partly because of their low-fat, plant-based meals, and partly because they are more physically active, a factor we will discuss shortly.

Animal fat holds a huge load of calories that does nothing good for the body and does a lot of harm, from promoting heart disease to increasing cancer risk, and, of course, fattening you up. Take a look at the fat content of various foods in Table 1, which is listed as a percentage of calories, rather than by weight. This is a critical difference. Whole milk, for example, is 3.3 percent fat by weight, because it is loaded with water. But when you drink it, your body separates out the water. The remaining milk solids contain a lot of fat--contributing 49 percent of milk's calories, to be exact. Milk that is two percent fat by weight is actually about 35 percent fat as a percentage of calories. It is actually not a low-fat product at all.

Table I

COMPARE THE FAT: PLANT VERSUS ANIMAL PRODUCTS

PLANT PRODUCTS	ANIMAL PRODUCTS
Baked beans (vegetarian) 4%	Beef (sirloin) 38%
Black beans 4%	Beef (top round) 29%
Broccoli 8%	Catfish 33%
Butternut squash 2%	Chicken, white, skinless 23%
Cantaloupe 6%	Cottage cheese, "2%" 20%
Carrots 3%	Egg, fresh 64%
Cauliflower 6%	Halibut 19%
Cream of Wheat 4%	Lamb, lean 34%
Creamed corn 5%	Milk, whole 49%
Orange 1%	Milk, "2%" 35%
Peas 3%	Salmon, Atlantic 40%
Potato <1%	Swordfish 30%
Rice <1%	Tuna 16%
Spaghetti noodles 4%	Turkey, oven-roasted 21%
Spinach 7%	Venison, lean 29%

Figures given are percentages of calories from fat.
Source: J.A.T. Pennington. Bowes and Church's Food Values of Portions Commonly Used. (New York: Harper and Row, 1989).

McDonald's advertises its McLean DeLuxe burger as "91 percent fat-free," meaning that, by weight, it is nine percent fat. But as a percentage of calories, which is what dietitians care about, the McLean DeLuxe patty is 49 percent fat, hardly something anyone would recommend. Even the so-called "lean" cuts of beef are nowhere near the truly low-fat foods--beans, grains, vegetables, and fruits--most of which are less than 10% fat. The problem with meats, including poultry and fish, is that they are muscles, and muscles are made up of protein and fat.

Advertisers sometimes claim that chicken is a low-fat food. Is it? No matter how chicken is prepared, it cannot get its calorie level down to that of the truly healthful foods, because chicken, like all meats, is permeated with fat. So while beans and rice are just four percent and one percent fat, respectively, chicken is over 20 percent fat, even after the skin is removed.

Some people eat fish in the hope that the omega-3 fatty acids in fish oils will reduce their cholesterol levels. Actually, fish oils may reduce triglycerides somewhat, but do not reduce cholesterol levels and do not prevent heart problems. When Harvard researchers studied the heart attack rate in 44,895 male health professionals, they found that those who ate the most fish actually ended up with more heart problems than those who rarely ate fish.[14] Happily, the negative calorie effect foods are terrific for weight loss and reducing cholesterol levels. Since they are plant-derived, they contain no cholesterol at all.

Fish oils are just as fattening as any other fat or oil, with nine calories in every gram. While most fish are similar to other animal products in fat content, some are lower, but this does not even begin to make them recommended foods. Remember, fish contains no complex carbohydrates and no fiber, and tends to displace these foods from the meal. As mentioned above, low-carbohydrate diets tend to encourage the inactivation of thyroid hormone, so they do not help your metabolism one bit. All fish products also contain cholesterol, and the protein they contain can contribute to other problems, as we will see shortly.

In summary, meats, poultry, and fish have two main problems for those concerned about their weight. First, like all muscles, they have inherent fat with its concentrated calories. Second, because muscle tissues are mainly just protein and fat, they displace the complex carbs that are essential to the negative calorie effect. So the first prescription for cutting the fat is the V-word: vegetarian foods are, by far, the most powerful foods for weight control. As you have probably heard, vegetarian foods have also shown their power to help reverse heart disease, prevent cancer, and make diabetes and high blood pressure much more manageable and, in some cases, disappear entirely.

Back at Bill and Susan's house, our friends are in the kitchen whipping up some tacos. Or, to be more precise, Bill is clowning around in a sombrero he bought in Cancun, while Susan is comparing two different recipes for taco filling. One is made with ground beef and the other uses beans. Ground beef is about 60 percent fat, and three ounces of ground beef hold about 225 calories. Beans are very low in fat--less than 5 per-cent--and three ounces hold only about 80 calories. So by ig-noring Bill's advice and choosing the bean recipe instead, Susan reduces the calories in their tacos by nearly two-thirds.

Vegetable Oils

Vegetable oils have a good reputation because they contain no cholesterol and are low in saturated fats. That makes them a much healthier choice for your heart than animal fats. But as far as their calorie content goes, they are the same as any other kind of fat.

For example, a potato is very modest in calories, and only about one percent fat. When it is baked, no extra oil is added. But if it is cut into french fries and dropped into cooking oil, its fat content soars up to 47 percent, and its calorie content nearly triples. Similarly, compare the fat content of a doughnut (50%), which is fried in oil, to a bagel (8%), which is not. The dough-nut ends up with more than six times the fat!

Fat on your plate adds easily to your body fat. Unlike carbo-hydrates, which lose nearly a quarter of their calories if your body tries to make fat from them, fats and oils in foods can in-sinuate their way onto your hips or thighs almost unchanged.

They cause other problems, too. Fat in foods increases the risk of several forms of cancer (breast, colon, prostate and oth-ers), heart disease, diabetes, gallstones, and other serious con-ditions. Although animal fats are the worst, vegetable oils also contribute to health problems.

We do need a tiny amount of fat in the diet. But we need only a fraction of what most of us typically get. A small amount of fat is inherent in grains, legumes, and vegetables. This is all the body needs. Children can (and perhaps should) have a bit more fat in their diet. Breast milk is naturally higher in fat for the needs of growing infants. The natural process of weaning eliminates this nutrient when it is no longer appropriate.

Rick: Swearing Off Grease

Rick worked in the computer room at a university, and potato chips, buttered popcorn, peanut butter, chicken, and onion rings were all part of the lunch room routine. He had been fairly slim until he reached about 25, when his waistline gradually began to expand. At 40, he was about 30 pounds overweight. His daily intake of fatty foods had had a predictable effect.

He tried low-calorie diets, but found he couldn't stick to them. So he signed up at a commercial weight loss center in a mall near his home, figuring it would work better. But it became rather expensive and really did not work much better than diets he had tried on his own.

He read about the approach described in this book, and felt it made sense. Although he was not sure that he wanted to change his menu forever, he tried it as a three-week experiment. There was no limit on amounts, but he was very strict to omit oils, margarine, salad dressings, and all meats and dairy products. After three weeks, he had lost seven pounds. That was a good start, and he also found that he had lost all desire for greasy foods, and began to associate them with his weight problems. So he decided to stick with his new way of eating for three more weeks. He lost five more pounds. A month later, he had lost another five pounds, and his weight loss continued until he reached the weight he had in college. His girlfriend used the same method to drop from 155 to 120 pounds.

People at work started to notice the change in his eating habits and in how he looked. His co-worker Mike, who weighed 275 pounds, decided to try this approach, too, and lost 80 pounds.

Getting Free from the Fat in Foods

A low-fat menu is a recipe for a slim, healthy body. The most powerful weight-control menus cut out animal products completely and keep vegetable oils to a minimum, too. Of course, it does take some getting used to. Unfortunately, grease is almost like an addicting substance. For the first month or so after you cut chicken, burgers, potato chips, and onion rings out of your diet, you will have a tendency to want to return to them, so be on the look-out. It is actually easier to cut them out entirely than to continually tease yourself with them occasionally. Later on, I'll share with you some tips and plenty of recipes to make it easy.

Fat Substitutes

Chemical fat substitutes have recently emerged. Simplesse, made by the NutraSweet Company, is made of a protein that simulates the texture of grease on the tongue. Because it changes consistency when heated, Simplesse can only be used in foods which are not baked or fried. Olestra is a sucrose polyester made by Procter and Gamble. It is designed to taste and feel like fat, but is indigestible and unabsorbable.

I find it impossible to be enthusiastic about these products. Like chemical sweeteners, their safety remains in doubt. Some contend that Olestra may cause cancer and liver problems. In addition, they reinforce the taste for fat, rather than help you break the grease habit.

WHAT ABOUT ALCOHOL?

In general, health recommendations have been mixed on alcohol. Modest alcohol consumption--one to two drinks per day--may slightly reduce the risk of heart problems. On the other hand, even small amounts of alcohol increase the risk of breast cancer and contribute to birth defects. And, of course, beyond modest use, alcohol contributes to many other very serious health problems, from accidents to heart disease, cancer, nerve

disorders, and digestive problems.
What about its effect on your waistline? This is no mystery.
Alcohol is fattening. People who consume beer, wine, or mixed
drinks on a regular basis get a big load of extra calories.

Calories in Alcoholic Beverages

Wine (4 oz.)	85
Light Beer (12 oz.)	100
Beer (12 oz.)	150
Liquor, 100 proof (1.5 oz.)	124

What is important about alcohol, however, is not just its calorie content. The important point is this: Alcohol <u>adds</u> to the
calories you are already consuming, rather than displacing any.
For example, if you were to eat four bread sticks before dinner,
you would eat a bit less at dinner. The 150 calories' worth of
bread would displace about the same amount from the food you
would have later. But alcohol does not seem to follow this
compensatory mechanism. If you substitute a beer for the bread
sticks, it also holds 150 calories, and these calories are not nec-
essarily compensated for by eating less later. The calories in
alcohol <u>add</u> to them. Even worse, alcohol can slow down your
calorie-burning speed.[15,16]

SWEETS AND SWEETENERS

Concentrated sugars, such as hard candies, are just chunks of
the simplest form of carbohydrate, with the natural fiber and
water removed. As a result, they are as concentrated a form of
calories as can be found in a carbohydrate food. If you consume large quantities of sugary foods, such as sweets and sodas,
you will get more calories than your body needs. Even so, sugars are not nearly as calorie-dense as fats. If you are not controlling the amount of fat you are eating, there is little point in
worrying about sugar.

Often, sugar is not the main problem in sweets. In cookies,

pies, and cakes, there is usually a huge amount of fat, too. Of the 540 calories in a cup of Haagen-Dazs vanilla ice cream, 57 percent are from fat. Fifty percent of the calories in a Hershey dark chocolate bar are from fat. A modest serving of Pillsbury German chocolate cake holds 250 calories, 40 percent of which are from fat. Two Chips Ahoy cookies hold 130 calories, 42 percent of which are from fat. When selecting sweet foods, pick those with the lowest amount of fat. How about fruit for desert?

Forget artificial sweeteners. They are no answer to weight problems. First of all, they are no substitute for using the real factors that you have learned about in this book. Second, what are you really gaining? Using an artificial sweetener instead of a teaspoon of sugar saves you only 16 calories. But just two grams of fat hold more calories than that. This is not to say that you should load up on sugar, but artificial sweeteners are a distraction from the real dietary issues, which for most people relate to the overload of fat and the lack of complex carbs and fiber in the foods they eat.

More importantly, sweeteners can have risks. Evidence links aspartame (NutraSweet) to a variety of effects on the brain. Headaches are common, and there is currently a scientific debate over whether it can cause grand mal seizures in adults or other brain effects in children, including babies developing in the womb. While the toxicologists fight it out, I see no special value in chemical sweeteners.

WHAT ABOUT GENETICS?

Some people may believe that, because genetics influences our size and shape, there is nothing they can do to lose weight. Not true. Although traits are passed from parents to children, they are simply tendencies; they do not seal your fate.[17] Also, we do not just give our children DNA. We also give them recipes. We give them preferences for various kinds of food. We also pass along our values about physical activity, health, and how our bodies should look. In other words, what we may assume to be due to assume to be due to genetics may be the result of food habits and attitudes passed down from generation to generation. They can be changed if we decide to do so. Whatever hand we have been dealt by our inheritance, there are still steps we can take to change our weight.

We tend to inherit our parents' shape. If your parents were apple-shaped, carrying their weight in their chests and abdomens, you are likely to be apple-shaped as well. If they were "pears," with most of their weight in their hips and thighs, you are likely to be a bit pear-shaped, too. There are all sorts of shape variations. Size is more easily changed than shape. If you carry your weight in your hips, as you lose weight you might become a skinny "pear," but you may still be a "pear."

Measure Your Health Risks

Waistline fat is easier to lose than hip fat. Losing it is a good idea because it is more likely than hip or thigh fat to contribute to health problems, including heart disease, cancer, diabetes, high blood pressure, and many others. To determine whether you are at greater risk for health problems from being overweight, measure around your waist and your hips at the widest points.

Men: Increased risk begins when your waist is bigger than your hips.

Women: Health risks begin when your waist is more than 80 percent of your hip measurement.

If you have passed your risk point, your weight problem is not just a cosmetic issue. It is a very real contributor to a broad range of health problems that you do not want.

SUMMARY OF BASIC CONCEPTS

Let's review the basics we've covered so far. The negative calorie effect comes from foods that are high in carbohydrate and low in fat: grains, beans, vegetables, and fruits. Complex carbs cannot add directly to your body fat, and they increase your calorie-burning ability. Taking advantage of their benefits while avoiding fats and oils is a powerful combination.

The best approach is to avoid animal products, as they never have any complex carbs or fiber, and they are typically high in fat. Keep vegetable oil, refined sugars, and alcohol to a minimum as well.

There is no need to limit the amount you eat, unless you are eating well past the point when you are full.

Also, there is no need to decide to change your eating habits for the rest of your life. That's more of a commitment than you need. Just try it for three weeks, and if you like it, you can stick with it. But to get the results you want, do not water down these guidelines. Adding occasional servings of chicken or french fries will slow your progress and will lure you back to the unhealthy foods that cause so many weight problems. Give yourself the best.

CHECK YOUR KNOWLEDGE

Try these questions. You'll find the answers below.

1. Carbohydrate-rich foods are vital for long-term weight control. In each pair, which has more carbohydrate?
   a. A fish fillet or broccoli
   b. Bread or beef
   c. Milk or a potato
   d. Cheese or rice

2. For each pair below, see if you can pick which is lower in fat.
   a. Fried chicken or broiled top round beef
   b. Leanest beef or leanest chicken
   c. Leanest chicken or vegetarian baked beans
   d. Leanest beef or rice
   e. Leanest chicken or a potato
   f. Spaghetti with tomato sauce or a <u>Lean Cuisine</u> spaghetti with meatballs dinner
   g. Baked potato or french fries
   h. A doughnut or a bagel

ANSWERS:

1. The numbers given are percentages of calories from carbohydrate:
   a. The difference is like day and night. Broccoli is 78% carbohydrate. Fish has no carbohydrate at all.
   b. Easy, isn't it? Bread is 75% carbohydrate. Beef has no carbohydrate at all.
   c. A potato is 93% carbohydrate. Milk is 30% carbohydrate, in the form of simple sugar.
   d. Rice has much more carbohydrate(89%) than cheese(1%).

2. The numbers given are percentages of calories from fat:
   a. Broiled top round beef (38%) is lower in fat than fried chicken (50% fat), but both are high-fat foods.
   b. Skinless chicken breast is about 20% fat,and lower than the leanest beef (29% fat), although both are high in fat compared to grains, beans, vegetables, and fruits.
   c. No contest. Vegetarian baked beans (4% fat) are much lower in fat than even the very leanest chicken (about 20%).
   d. Rice (less than 1%) has much less fat than the leanest beef (29% fat).
   e. A potato (1%) is far lower in fat than the leanest chicken (20% fat).
   f. Spaghetti with tomato sauce (6%) has only a fraction of the fat in a Lean Cuisine spaghetti with meatballs dinner (23%).
   g. A baked potato (1%) has much less fat than french fries (47%).
   h. A bagel (8%) is much lower in fat than a dough-nut (50%).

3

COMPULSIVE EATING AND CRAVINGS

Most overweight people do not overeat. Many actually eat <u>less</u> than thin people do, and their weight problems have more to do with the type of food they eat than the amount. But some people do tend to keep eating long after others have had enough. If you find yourself in this situation, you can learn what to do about it.

As we saw earlier, one big reason for overeating is the restrained-eater phenomenon, which simply means binges that kick in after periods of very-low-calorie dieting. They can affect anyone, even people who have never had a tendency to binge before or to overeat for any psychological reason. The key, of course, is to avoid the very-low-calorie diets that lead to binges.

EATING IN RESPONSE TO EMOTIONS

Some people eat when they are under stress. Depression, anxiety, hurt feelings, anger, or sadness are answered with a trip to the kitchen. Ask yourself these questions:

* Is food your usual answer to stress, anger, or sadness?
* Do you eat differently when others are around than when you are alone?
* Do you hide food?
* Do you eat when you are not at all hungry?
* Do you snack throughout the day?
* Do you order more than one entree at a restaurant?

If the answer to any of these is yes, then this section may be for you. Do not feel that you need to plumb the depths of your psyche and rearrange its contents in short order. For now, you need to make a plan to compensate for the tendency to eat in response to emotions.

Anticipate that from time to time, like it or not, you will become angry or sad or frustrated with things, and plan to deal with these feelings in another way. Is there someone you can talk to, or someone you can call? If food is a comfort, what other comforts can you take advantage of? For example, are there certain places, photographs, books, or clothes that serve as comforts, too? A long walk by a lake or other nature spot may help, as may going to a gym.

Deal with emotions in ways that are inconsistent with eating. For example, if you plan to get together with a friend, be with someone who is not preoccupied with eating, and pick a place where eating will not occur--meet in a park or office instead of a restaurant. As mealtime approaches, fill up on healthful foods first.

Are you eating out of boredom? We need many forms of nourishment: friends, intellectual challenges, physical activities, romance, challenges and successes in our lives, rest, and sleep. When these are absent, food may become a cheap substitute. Is food taking the place of something else?

If you are saying, "I overeat, but I do it because food tastes so good," it may be worth examining what else occupies your time. If your life is filled with boredom, then food may well be the most exciting thing in it. It is important to see what prevents you from engaging more fully in other activities that make life what it is.

Here are two keys to beating compulsive eating: First, build your menu from grains, beans, vegetables and fruits without added oils. These foods tend not to encourage weight gain, even when you sometimes overdo it. Let's say you have a slip. If your kitchen is stocked with these healthy foods, that slip is not nearly so likely to affect your weight.

Second, Overeaters Anonymous is a support group that meets regularly in nearly every city and can help you break out of compulsive eating. It is free and has helped many, many people. Check your local telephone directory.

The combination of a plant-based diet and the support of OA can get you well on your way to coping with the emotional roller coasters of life without plunging into self-destructive habits, and even to smoothing out the ups and downs a bit.

QUIETING YOUR CRAVINGS

Do chocolates, candies, fried snacks, or other foods call to you irresistibly, making you dash to the refrigerator or the store, mowing down anyone in your path? It can be a very uncomfortable feeling when foods take on that much power, especially if they happen to be very fattening foods. We would be healthier if we were to have an overwhelming urge for broccoli on a regular basis, but we are more likely to lunge for cream-filled donuts. If cravings lead you to foods that you would rather avoid, let me show you some ways to manage them.

It helps to understand what cravings are. If you were to go without water for a day or two, you would begin to crave water. If you were to go without air for even several seconds, you would crave air. A craving is a signal that your body sends to your brain that you need something--air, water, or food--to survive, and you need it soon. It is part of your body's system for balancing its physical needs.

It makes sense that your body would respond to a lack of water or air with a sense of urgency. But although it may sometimes feel like it, a lack of chocolate is not really life-threatening. So why do we crave chocolate?

Our internal balancing and signaling systems were established millions of years ago, long before the sun had set on the Stone Age. In very early human history, starvation was a real possibility, and our bodies had built-in systems to increase our hunger during times of famine. Our sense of thirst guided us to have more water when needed. But there were no chocolate donuts. Pure sugar sources were rare indeed. There were no fried foods until concentrated oils were developed and fire was available to heat them up. Cro-Magnon man did call out for cheese pizza--no one milked cows until much later in history. Coffee, alcohol, and cigarettes did not yet exist.

The foods and drinks we crave, in nearly every case, were not part of human experience until fairly recently, from a historical standpoint. We have no good built-in balancing systems for dealing with them. So while our bodies know exactly when to take in air and water, and exactly how much, because our species, like all animals, has been using them since time immemorial, we have no built-in means of coping with chocolate, coffee, potato chips, or alcohol.

Food cravings can represent three things:

1. Some foods can turn on our taste buds so strongly that they are hard to resist. Typically, these are foods that were not around when human taste buds first developed.

2. Some parts of our meals, such as caffeine and alcohol, are physically addicting. Cravings for them are part of the withdrawal symptoms that begin several hours after the last dose. Some people have suggested that chocolate may also be physically habituating. Whether that is true is not yet known, but chocolate does contain several chemicals that affect the brain, as we will see shortly.

3. A craving may represent a false signal. For example, your body may actually need a nutrient, but it signals you for something different. Some researchers believe that chocolate cravings are fueled by a lack of magnesium. In that case, it is the magnesium in chocolate that your body needs, not chocolate itself.

Identify Your Craving Profile

Different people are drawn to different foods. Women are more often drawn to chocolate, while men tend to have a taste for fried and greasy foods. Time of day and social circumstances can have important effects, too. It helps to understand the characteristics of your cravings, so you can anticipate them and decide what to do about them.

One important point: If your cravings are not causing you a health problem or increasing your weight and they are not escalating, then you may not need to worry about them. It is only when they are leading you in a dangerous direction that you need be concerned.

If you crave a fattening food regularly, I would suggest setting aside the guilty feelings that many people experience. Think of it, instead, as one of many fattening foods that people are challenged with, and you can plan what to do about it without making it a big moral issue.

If you are trying to tone down your cravings, first make sure your daily menu contains the foods you need to keep your satiety trigger working properly. That is your natural feeling of having had enough to eat, and it depends on eating plenty of complex carbs every day. They help normalize your appetite. Many people report that their cravings diminish when they improve their menus.

It also helps to eat regularly, rather than miss meals. For most people, that means three meals a day or perhaps more. As you know by now, skipping meals invites cravings and binges.

Regular physical activity helps, too. It tends to regularize your appetite and helps you sleep better so you feel more like taking care of yourself.

Common Cravings

Let's take a look at the most commonly craved foods and what to do about them:

Chocolate is, by far, the most frequently craved food, particularly for women, but also for many men. Its sugary taste and creamy texture seduce the taste buds. Regrettably, a typical chocolate bar has about 15 grams of fat. That is a lot. It would take, believe it or not, 75 cups of rice or 150 potatoes to match that amount.

Notice how chocolate affects the way you feel. Like all high-sugar foods, it can cause irritability or depressed moods, because of sugar's effect on brain chemistry. In addition, chocolate contains a substance called phenylethylamine, or PEA, which is chemically similar to amphetamines, drugs that are sometimes called "speed." A bit of PEA is produced in your body naturally whether you eat chocolate or not. In fact, some researchers believe that, in social situations when we are praised or applauded, a rush of PEA leads to the feeling of elation and high energy we experience. Rejection, they believe, causes a slow-down of PEA production, leading to low energy, increased sleep, and overeating.[18] Researchers speculate that some people eat chocolate to boost their moods by restoring the PEA their bodies lack. If it does act like amphetamines, it is worth noting that amphetamines can cause paranoid symptoms after prolonged use. Both chocolate and PEA can also cause migraines in susceptible people.[19]

Why is chocolate so "addicting"? Researchers have attributed this to its sugar or its creamy texture, or to various chemicals it contains--caffeine, theobromine, and magnesium, in addition to PEA.

If chocolate has become a problem for you, you can reduce the amount by using it as a flavoring for other foods, like chocolate-covered strawberries or bananas, rather than as a solid block. Some brands of cocoa powder, such as Hershey's, are less fatty than chocolate itself and can be used in cooking.

To reduce chocolate cravings, some physicians recommend magnesium supplements (300 milligrams twice a day).[20] They are available at health food stores. Also, the antidepressant bupropion (Wellbutrin) has been shown to knock out chocolate cravings for some people.[21] Bupropion's chemical structure is similar to PEA.

Sugary Foods- are not likely to cause weight problems unless you persistently overdo it, although they can cause depression, irritability, or fatigue for some people. However, when sweet cookies, cakes, and pies are made with a fair amount of fat, they really can expand your waistline.

If you do find yourself overdoing it on sweets, you might try increasing the amount of grains or other starchy foods on your menu. Starches break down to natural simple sugars in your body. Sometimes a sweet tooth can be a part of carbohydrate craving, which we will address next.

Carbohydrate Craving- Some people have a particular craving for carbohydrates. It is not because of their taste--the foods can be either sweet or starchy--but rather, due to the way carbohydrates affect brain chemistry. Carbohydrates boost a brain chemical called <u>serotonin</u>, which is important in brain functions, including sleep and mood regulation. Most antidepressants increase the amount of serotonin in the brain, among other actions. Carbohydrate cravers experience frequent depressions, particularly in the winter months when the days are short. They eat high-carb foods because they have noticed that they help them feel better, presumably by increasing the amount of serotonin in the brain.

There is nothing wrong with eating generous amounts of carbohydrates. The key is to select foods rich in <u>complex</u> carbohydrates, such as rice and other grains, beans, and vegetables, rather than sugar candies, and to avoid sugar-fat mixtures, like cakes, cookies, and doughnuts, which tend to be fattening.

There are treatments for mid-winter depressions and the cravings that come with them. For example, special high-intensity lights are used in the morning and evening to improve moods. Some antidepressants help diminish cravings, although others actually seem to cause them, which can necessitate a change of medication.

Fried or Greasy Foods- Many people crave potato chips, onion rings, and other greasy foods. If that includes you, it really helps to reset your grease "set-point." The amount of fat we consume tends to stay fairly constant from one day to the next. You can reset your taste for fat by conscientiously and drastically reducing the amount for about three weeks. The results can be very surprising.

As you know, getting away from animal products and vegetable oils is the most powerful strategy for weight control. It does require a bit of self-control at first, but you will soon find that you want much less fat in your foods. You many well find yourself turned off by greasy foods, and will appreciate the benefits that remain long afterward.

Meats- Meats are often craved for a while by people who are trying to get away from all that fat and cholesterol. That makes sense, since they are among the most calorie-dense foods people eat. Happily, meat substitutes typically cure the meat-craving very quickly. See the selection at your health food store. Choose those lowest in fat, and experiment with different brands.

Cheese- Some cheeses (and sausage) contain even more PEA than is in chocolate. Is that why cheese can be so addicting? No one knows, but cheese is certainly among the most waist-line-padding foods.

For a great cheese taste with none of the disadvantages of dairy products, try the Cheesy Garbanzo Spread in the recipe section. It is much lower in fat than typical cheeses, although not so low as the other recipes. You might also try sprinkling some nutritional yeast flakes on pizza or sauces. It has a cheesy taste and is available at all health food stores.

When Do Cravings Hit?

Let's identify which circumstances make you most vulnerable to cravings:

Hunger- Some cravings are intensified by hunger. The solution is to eat regular meals and, if a craving does kick in, have something healthy to eat to reduce hunger.

Fatigue- If your cravings tend to come when you are tired, see what you can do to get more rest. Regular exercise also tends to help.

Before or During Periods- Women in their twenties often find that food cravings occur during their menstrual periods.[22]

Women in their thirties or forties often find that cravings cluster the week before their period. Understanding when you are vulnerable may help you cope.

Reducing your fat intake can also influence menstrual changes. A lower fat intake reduces the amount of estrogen your body produces during your monthly cycle and seems to make both the physical and psychological changes at the end of the month much less dramatic. In fact, women who switch to a low-fat, vegetarian diet often report that their cramps diminish markedly.

Researchers have found that women with premenstrual syndrome (PMS) are sometimes low in magnesium.[23] This may help account for chocolate cravings, since chocolate is loaded with magnesium.

Spicy Foods and Alcohol- If spicy foods send you racing down the chocolate highway, you might try experimenting with less piquant fare or have a sweet orange standing by for the end of the meal.

Alcohol, of course, can compromise just about any resolve. By now, you know whether it affects you in this way.

Evenings- are the time when cravings tend to hit hardest. Make sure you've had a good dinner, so you are not hungry, and keep healthy snacks on hand.

Satisfying a craving is not the end of the world. Most people have them. If your menu is generally healthy, the occasional sugary indulgence is not going to be a problem, unless it escalates. If cravings are guiding you toward fattening foods and ruining your progress, you can use these tips to help you.

4

ASSURING COMPLETE NUTRITION

Foods with the negative calorie effect are nutritious for all stages of life--childhood, adulthood, pregnancy, nursing, menopause, and older age. But with any change in your diet, you will want to assure that you get all the nutrients your body needs. Happily, this is very easy to do.

PROTEIN

Before the 1980's, many people believed that it was difficult to get complete protein on plant-based diets. We now know that it is actually very simple. As the American Dietetic Association states, a varied menu of plant foods easily provides enough protein, even without any special combining.[24] As long as you get even a modest variety, you will have no trouble.

It was also commonly believed that the more protein in your diet, the better. We now know different. High-protein diets are actually risky, encouraging the loss of calcium from the body and overworking the kidneys.

The bone-thinning disease of osteoporosis is an epidemic in Western countries, and animal protein is an important part of its cause. This has been shown repeatedly in scientific studies. Yale University researchers recently found that the more meat people eat in various countries, the more fractures they tend to have, a sign of the bone-weakening effect of animal protein.[25] Likewise, when researchers feed animal protein to volunteers and then test their urine a little later, they find that bone calcium ends up in their urine.

A protein molecule is like a string of beads, and each "bead" is an amino acid molecule. When you digest proteins, these amino acids make your blood slightly acidic. Scientists believe that it is in the process of buffering this acid that calcium is pulled from the bones. Ultimately, it is discarded in the urine. In addition, meat protein is very high in what are called "sulfur-containing amino acids," which are suspected of being particularly likely to leach calcium from the bones. Switching from beef to chicken or fish does not help, because they have as much animal protein as beef, or even more. On the other hand, when you eliminate meat, cheese and eggs from your meals, your calcium losses can be cut in half.[26]

Although many of us grew up being taught to make sure we got enough protein, the fact is, we have gotten too much. There is adequate protein in beans, grains, and vegetables. But meats and eggs contain much more protein than the body can use. That excess protein not only interferes with the calcium balance of the body. It can also overwork the kidneys. Excess amino acids and their byproducts act as diuretics, forcing the kidneys to work harder than they should. The nephrons, which are the kidneys' filter units, slowly die off in the process.

The gradual loss of calcium and of kidney function can occur, not just in those who consume high-protein formulas, but in anyone who consumes meat, chicken, or fish on a regular basis. The best advice about protein is to stick with plant sources. Any normal variety of grains, beans, and vegetables will do the job. There is no need to carefully combine proteins from different plant sources. But when meats are included, the protein content easily becomes more than the body can handle safely. For example, if you were to have a single seven-ounce serving of roast beef, you would get 62 grams of protein. This one serving contains more than the recommended dietary allowance of protein for a whole day. Including such foods forces protein intake into the danger zone.

Let's take a look at two other high-protein products: egg whites and skim milk. Doctors learned long ago that egg yolks were loaded with cholesterol. A single egg yolk contains 213 mg of cholesterol (and is 80% fat). That is even more cholesterol than in an eight-ounce steak. But while many doctors now recommend avoiding egg yolks, some still encourage the consumption of egg whites because they contain protein. Well, the fact is that two eggs give you fully 12 grams of animal protein, a huge amount that no one needs.

Skim milk is a similar wrong turn. Because of the high saturated fat content of whole milk, many people have chosen skim dairy products. Getting rid of the dairy fat is certainly a good idea, because the fat in whole milk, butter, cheese, cream, and ice cream can increase the risk of heart disease and cancer, in addition to affecting your waistline. But after the fat is removed, skim milk is hardly a health food. It has no fiber and no complex carbs, and its calories come from two things you definitely do not need--lactose sugar (55 percent of calories) and animal proteins (about 40 percent of calories).

If you thought you needed milk for strong bones, you have been the victim of an extremely aggressive advertising program by the dairy industry which was not based on good science. You will find more on how to keep your bones healthy in the next section.

Some weight loss regimens emphasize high-protein foods and use very little carbohydrate. They load you up with chicken, fish, eggs, etc., hoping for a rapid water loss. But usually the weight comes back on very quickly, and such diets are far from healthful.

CALCIUM

For calcium, two issues are important: first, holding on to the calcium you have in your bones already and, second, including calcium in your diet to make up for natural losses.

Osteoporosis is a serious problem, particularly for women after menopause. But the cause is not usually an inadequate calcium intake. The problem is abnormally rapid loss of calcium from the bones. Factors that affect this calcium drain have been identified, and they might surprise you.

* As noted above, animal protein is a major culprit in the loss of calcium from bones, and avoiding animal protein completely can cut calcium losses in half.[26]

* Salt encourages calcium loss via the kidneys. Cutting your salt intake in half can reduce your calcium needs substantially.[27]

* Go easy on the caffeine. If you limit your caffeine intake to no more than two cups of coffee per day, your bones will have an easier time holding on to calcium.[28] Use decaf, or try one of the coffee substitutes sold in health food stores.

* Don't smoke. Long-term smokers have ten percent weaker bones, compared to nonsmokers. That ten percent difference can spell a 44 percent increase in the risk of a hip fracture.[29]

* Regular physical activity helps keep your bones strong, while sedentary living weakens them.

* Your bones also like a little sun. As sunlight touches the skin, it turns on the natural production of vitamin D, which helps keep your bones strong. Brief periods of sun exposure on a regular basis can give your body all the vitamin D it needs.

* If you rarely see the sun, you will need supplemental vitamin D, which is in all multiple vitamins. Any common brand containing 5-10 micrograms (200-400 IU), taken daily, provides adequate vitamin D.[30] Avoid higher doses. By the way, the vitamin D added to some milk products is not natural to milk. It is simply a vitamin supplement added by the dairy, sometimes with insufficient attention to how much or how little is added.

You do need calcium in your diet. But don't depend on a high calcium intake to protect your bones if you are not controlling the calcium-depleters listed above. Many research studies have shown that calcium intake has little effect on osteoporosis, particularly at the hip and spine.[31-34] The Yale researchers mentioned above found that, contrary to what one might expect, countries with higher calcium consumption actually had more hip fractures, not fewer.[25] Calcium does not cause the fractures. Rather, calcium is simply too weak to counteract the effect of the high protein intake caused by the meat-and-dairy diet in Western countries. The fact is, you can keep strong bones with a much more modest calcium intake when you avoid the calcium-depleters. Of course, if you get very little calcium, say less than 400 milligrams per day, you may not be giving your body the calcium it needs.[32,34]

The healthiest calcium sources are green leafy vegetables and legumes or, as some people say, "greens and beans." A cup of broccoli has 178 milligrams of calcium, and it comes in a more absorbable form than the calcium in milk.[35] Beans and other legumes are also loaded with calcium. You don't need to eat huge servings of broccoli or beans to get enough calcium, but do include both in your regular menu planning.

If you are looking for a source of extra calcium, fortified orange juice is a good choice. It contains calcium citrate, which is much more readily absorbed than the calcium in milk or in calcium carbonate supplements.[36]

HEALTHFUL CALCIUM SOURCES (MILLIGRAMS)

Black beans (1 cup, boiled)	103	Lentils (1 cup, boiled)	37
Broccoli (1 cup, boiled)	178	Navel orange (1 medium)	56
Brussels sprouts (8 sprouts)	56	Navy beans (1 cup, boiled)	128
Butternut squash (1 cup, boiled)	84	Onions (1 cup, boiled)	58
Chick peas (1 cup, canned)	78	Orange juice, calcium-fortified (1 cup)*	300
Collards (1 cup, boiled)	148	Pancake mix (1/4 cup, 3 pancakes)	140
Corn bread (1 2-ounce piece)	133	Pinto beans (1 cup, boiled)	82
English muffin	92	Soybeans (1 cup, boiled)	175
Figs, dried (10 medium)	269	Sweet potato (1 cup, boiled)	70
Great northern beans (1 cup, boiled)	121	Tofu (1/2 cup)	258

Green beans (1 cup, boiled)	58 Vegetarian baked beans (1 cup)	128
Kale (1 cup boiled)	94 Wax beans (1 cup, canned)	174
Kidney beans (1 cup, boiled)	50 Wheat flour, calcium enriched (1 cup)	238
White beans (1 cup, boiled)	161	

Source: J.A.T. Pennington, Bowes and Church's Food Values of Portions Commonly Used. (New York: Harper and Row, 1989.)

* package information

A WORD ABOUT B$_{12}$

One nutrient does deserve a bit of planning, although it is a very simple issue. Vitamin B$_{12}$ is needed in tiny amounts for healthy blood and healthy nerves. It is not made by plants or animals; it is made by bacteria and other microorganisms. Long ago, when our ancestors plucked vegetables from the ground, there were likely to be traces of B$_{12}$ on them, produced by the natural bacteria in the soil. The bacteria in their mouths may even have produced a trace of the vitamin. Modern hygiene and pasteurization have eliminated these sources. Meat-eaters get the vitamin B$_{12}$ produced by fecal bacteria in the intestinal tracts of animals, which passes into the animals' tissues, but, unfortunately, they get a load of fat and cholesterol along with it.

People who adhere to a vegetarian diet (as I recommend) should choose foods, such as breakfast cereals, that are supplemented with vitamin B$_{12}$ or pick up any common supplement. All common multivitamins (One-A-Day, Flintstones, StressTabs, etc.) contain B$_{12}$. The recommended dietary allowance is only two micrograms per day. Health food stores carry vegetarian brands which have the advantage of eliminating dairy and meat extracts. Your body stores a very good supply of this vitamin, but if you have been on a pure vegetarian diet for three years, you should begin taking any common supplement or include supplemented foods in your routine.

Many doctors now recommend vegetarian diets, because they have advantages that even lean-meat diets cannot touch. They are not just low in cholesterol. They have no cholesterol at all, and they are loaded with vitamins, minerals, and fiber, many of which are low or completely lacking in meats. Every day, we learn more about the advantages of plant-based diets, and it is now clear that they are optimal for human health.

Even so, it is always important--whatever diet you follow--to assure that you get all the nutrients your body needs.

CHECK YOUR KNOWLEDGE

Try each question. Answers are listed below.

1. How do alcoholic beverages affect weight problems?
2. What is the most fattening ingredient in pies and cookies?
3. True or false: Vegetarians get enough protein without carefully combining foods.
4. True or false: As far as protein is concerned, the more the better.
5. Pick the food in each pair which is lowest in fat:
   a. Spaghetti with meat sauce or spaghetti with tomato sauce
   b. A fast-food meat taco or a fast-food bean burrito
   c. Cheddar cheese or bread
   d. Peanut butter or rice
   e. Ice cream or jelly beans
6. What problems can be caused by diets with too much protein?

ANSWERS:

1. Alcohol holds plenty of calories, and may not reduce the amount of food eaten subsequently.
2. The fat in pies and cakes--in the form of shortening or butter--is much more fattening than whatever sugar they contain.
3. True. A varied diet of plant foods easily provides adequate protein.

4. False. We need some protein, and the amount in plant foods is sufficient, but adding high-protein products is not healthful.

5.
  a. Spaghetti with tomato sauce (6%) is much lower in fat than spaghetti with meat sauce (35%).
  b. A fast-food bean burrito (31%) is lower in fat than a fast-food meat taco (50%). Hold the cheese and it will be lower still.
  c. Bread (16%) has much less fat than cheddar cheese (74%). Most cheeses are extremely high in fat.
  d. Rice (less than 1%) is much lower in fat than peanut butter (78%).
  e. Jelly beans (less than 1%) are much lower in fat than ice cream (48%), although both hold a large amount of sugar.

6. Diets that are high in protein, especially animal protein, encourage osteoporosis and a gradual loss of kidney function.

LET'S GET STARTED

At this point, you have a good understanding of how the negative calorie effect works. Now it's time to put it into action. Give yourself a pat on the back. You wanted a change for the better, and here you are, well on your way there.

I am assuming that you want to get the most out of this program, so I will show you the very best way to proceed. Of course, any change--major or minor--in your eating habits can seem like a challenge at first. So here are a few tips that can make any transition easier.

1. Focus on exploration, rather than deprivation. It is fun to try new foods. Take a look at the astounding array of new cookbooks at your local bookstore, particularly those offering vegetarian cuisine, pastas, Mexican, Middle-eastern, or Asian foods, and on and on. They are a gold mine. Some use dairy products or more than minimal amounts of oil, but these recipes can usually be easily modified. If you have not already seen my other books, let me recommend them as a source of in-depth information on a broad range of health issues, as well as many delicious menus and recipes.

Exploring new food products can be delightful as well. Take a look at the health food store. You'll find a huge range of "transition foods"--healthy vegetarian substitutes for fatty, cholesterol-laden foods, like ice cream, mayonnaise, hot dogs, and hamburgers. Some may contain more vegetable oil than you will want, so choose those that are lowest in fat.   The range of new health food products is growing from one week to the next, from soups of every variety to dips and sandwich fillings to exotic dishes that are a snap to prepare.

When you try new recipes or new products, many will be terrific and a few will be duds. That's okay; it's what experimenting is all about. The idea is to be open to new ideas, new tastes, and new ways of thinking about your body.

2. Go for the best possible menu. Nothing is more encouraging than success, so go for the maximal reward. That means really following this program exactly. Weak menus get weak results.

3. Think short-term. There is no need to make plans about what you will do in the distant future. Just follow this program for three weeks. At the end of that time, see how you feel. Notice its effect on your waistline. And if you like what you see, you can try it again for another 21 days. If you continue, you will get its full benefit.

4. Do not tease yourself with unhealthy foods. Anyone who has tried to change a habit knows about this one. Take smoking, for example. If people only cut down on smoking, they get essentially nowhere, because the taste for tobacco stays in their minds. It is very easy to drift back into a habit that has not yet been fully broken. But if they quit completely, they can get some distance between themselves and tobacco and can get into the habit of being a non-smoker. The same is true of foods. If you have fried chicken or potato chips once a week, you are teasing yourself with these fattening products, and you will never lose your taste for them. If, however, you get away from them completely, you will allow your taste buds to learn a new habit.   You will get momentum working for you.

5. Involve your family and friends. Our families eat with us. They eat the food we make or, perhaps, make the food we eat. When researchers have worked with patients to improve their diets, they have found that their families can be a real asset. So ask them to support you in this program, and include them as you experiment with new ways of making lasagne, chili, soups, desserts, and other tasty foods. Now, they may not feel a need for any permanent change in their eating habits. And you do not need to ask them to change permanently. All you need to ask them to do is to join you while you are starting this program. They will benefit in the process. This new way of eating not only slims waistlines; it can also lower cholesterol levels, help control blood pressure, and help prevent cancer and many other serious conditions.

At the very least, however, ask your family and friends not to tempt you with unhealthful foods while you are revamping your menu, and do not prepare any unhealthful foods for them.

Families often get stuck in old habits. They may even want to talk you out of changing and may forecast failure. In that case, you need to have a short sit-down talk. Tell them that if they care about you, they will understand that this is very important to you. They will help and not hinder you. If you have done this with sufficient sincerity, they will be overcome with guilt and will plead for forgiveness. You might suggest that they can make it up to you by making your breakfast.

Help them to think of this program as simply experimenting with some new recipes.

Follow this program to the letter. You are embarking on a powerful and rewarding experience. Give it every chance for maximal success. You deserve no less, and I believe you will be really pleased with the results.

GETTING OFFENDING FOODS OUT OF THE HOUSE

It really helps to get rid of the fattening foods that have caused your weight problem and can get in your way in the future. They won't help you, they never have helped you, and it is best to be rid of them. You can throw them away or give them away, but the key is to get them out of the house. Then you can bring in foods that are powerful for permanent weight control.

Before you begin, have a meal. It is very difficult for a hungry person to throw any food product away, no matter how unhealthy it may be. Then go on a search-and-destroy mission for the high-fat, no-fiber foods in your house. Get rid of all of the following:

> Any meat, poultry, or fish products
> All salad dressings other than non-fat dressings
> All dairy products, including butter, milk or cream, yogurt, ice cream, and cheese
> Potato chips
> Margarine
> Cookies, cakes, and pies
> Vegetable oils and shortenings
> Nuts and nut butters
> Sugary candies

You may notice a certain sense of relief as you rid yourself of these unhealthful products. Now you can stock your shelves with foods that will help you get the body you want, using the menus and recipes in this book as your guide. Having a good supply of healthful foods eliminates the need for frequent shopping trips, which are times of vulnerability to impulse purchases.

I would suggest that you not go shopping on an empty stomach. If you do, you risk ending up buying buckets of ice cream, goofy fattening snacks, chocolate swirl-cake, and all the other seductions that greet hungry stomachs. Most of the foods you'll want are available from any grocery store, but a few are found at health food stores. Notice that you do not have to mix any diet powders or shop for special frozen dinners, and you never have to go hungry.

Making It Quick

Take a minute to leaf through the recipe section, which has many delicious breakfasts, sandwiches, soups, stews, main dishes, and desserts. All are designed for quick and easy preparation. Here are a few ideas for extra quick breakfasts, lunches, and dinners to get you out of the kitchen fast.

Quick Breakfast Ideas

* Fresh fruit: Melon, grapefruit, oranges, bananas, pineapple, or any other variety you like. Fruit can be your entire breakfast, or just the beginning.

* Hot cereal: Choose from old-fashioned oatmeal, Cream of Wheat, grits, or other hot cereal. Cooked versions are best, but instant is acceptable. Have it plain, or top it with cinnamon or jam, or try strawberries, raisins, or other fresh fruit. If you like to use milk, use soy or rice milk, which are not only free of animal fats; they are also free of the cholesterol, lactose, animal proteins, and contaminants that are found in dairy products. Low-fat varieties are best. Soy and rice milks are found at any health food store, or look near the condensed milks in the regular grocery.

* Whole-grain toast or bagels. Have them plain, or top with jam or cinnamon. Do not use butter, margarine, or cream cheese.

* Cold cereal with soy or rice milk. Choose whole-grain cereals, and top with fresh fruit if you like.

* For adventurous souls who like a hearty breakfast, try baked beans on toast. While this is almost unheard-of in North America, it is a breakfast tradition in Britain and Australia, where no restaurant would ever be without it. The Latin

American equivalent is black beans on toast. This breakfast sounds unusual, but can be popular on both sides of the border. Simply empty a can of baked beans or black beans into a saucepan and heat. Spoon the beans onto toast and, if you like, top with a touch of mild salsa or Dijon mustard. Middle-Eastern cuisine uses chickpeas (garbanzo beans) in much the same way, and they are as healthy they are quick. Just open a can of chick peas and rinse. Eat plain or with non-fat salad dressing. Try them! You'll be surprised.

Quick Lunch Ideas

At lunch time, convenience is often a key. Low-fat lunches not only help you slim down. They also prevent the after-lunch fatigue that follows high-fat meals.

* Instant soups. Health food stores and many regular groceries stock a beautiful variety, including split pea soup, noodle soups, couscous, and many others. You can keep them in your desk at work and just add hot water at lunchtime. If you prefer, bring a Thermos of vegetable soup or split pea from home.

* Check your natural food store for meatless "cold cuts." Made of soy or wheat, they are delicious in quick and easy sandwiches. Or have a CLT: cucumber, lettuce, and tomato on whole-grain bread. Add onion and mustard, if you like. Some people like to add sprouts, red or green peppers, or pickles. Unfortunately, most traditional sandwich fillings are loaded with fat. Among the problem foods are meats of any kind, cheese, mayonnaise, and peanut butter.

* Burritos are quick to make and very portable. They can be eaten hot or cold. Simply spread some fat-free refried pinto or black beans on a flour tortilla. (The word "refried" is a misnomer; they are actually boiled.) Add a bit of salsa and a salad for a delicious and satisfying meal, or use corn tortillas for "tacos to go."

* Keep a bag of prewashed salad mix and a jar of fat-free dressing on hand. Add some canned kidney beans or garbanzo beans for an almost-instant salad.

* How about a nice plate of <u>les</u> <u>Restes</u> <u>d'Hier</u>? That's what the French call leftovers. A bit of last night's dinner is always welcome, very fast, and microwavable.

* Fresh fruit: Enjoy bananas, apples, pears, oranges, strawberries, peaches, apricots, plums, tangerines, star fruit, raspberries, etc. Avoid avocados.

* Keep rice cakes, bread, bread sticks, pretzels, Melba toast, or carrot or celery sticks on hand for a quick complement to your meal. You can even find genuinely fat-free potato chips at health food stores.

* If you eat lunch in a cafeteria, enjoy the vegetables, potatoes, beans, breads, and the salad bar with a twist of lemon juice or a little vinegar and pepper instead of dressing. Avoid meats, eggs, and dairy products, and keep vegetable oils to an absolute minimum.

* Frozen grapes make a wonderful summertime snack. Simply remove them from the stems and freeze them, loosely packed, in an airtight container.

Quick Dinners

* Take a look at the recipe section in the back of this book. All are fast and easy to make. Pita Pizzas are especially quick. Serve them with commercially prepared three-bean salad. Other super-quick recipes include Pasta with Roasted Summer Vegetables, Quick Chili, Bean Tacos, Quick Pita Sandwiches, Black Bean Burritos, and Beanie Weenies.

* Chili keeps well in the refrigerator, and even improves over time as the spices get to know each other. It's ready to reheat when you are. Try my Super Chili recipe for a real treat. It is scrumptious on a bed of rice or spaghetti.

* Boxed curried rice or similar dinners keep on your shelf indefinitely and cook with almost no supervision.

* Frozen vegetables are very convenient, and their nutritional value is similar to that of fresh vegetables. Frozen veggies can also make recipes a snap. Instead of washing and chopping vegetables, you can buy frozen chopped onions, broccoli flo-

rets, carrots, cauliflower--you name it. While you're at it, you can buy crushed garlic in a jar. Just spoon out the amount you want. Of course, if you love to cook, you can always make recipes with fresh greens and real onions and garlic.

* For baked beans, black beans, or any other variety, buy them canned, rather than dried, and all you have to do is heat them up. Low-sodium versions are available at both regular groceries and health food stores. With potatoes or rice and some frozen vegetables, dinner's ready in a snap.

* Ramen soups are fast and delicious. Add some chopped fresh vegetables for a hearty soup (see the recipe section).

* Mix fat-free refried beans with an equal amount of salsa for a delicious bean dip. Serve with baked tortilla chips.

* Drain garbanzo beans and spoon into a piece of pita bread. Top with prewashed salad mix and fat-free salad dressing for a quick sandwich.

* Pick up some fat-free vegetarian burger patties at the health food store. There are so many varieties; see which ones you like best. For a super-quick meal, just pop one in the toaster oven or microwave. Serve it on a whole grain bun with mustard, ketchup, barbecue sauce, and lettuce. Add sliced red onion and tomato if desired.

* Keep pre-baked potatoes in the refrigerator. For a quick meal, heat one in the microwave and top it with chili, salsa, or Dijon mustard.

* Frozen bananas make a delicious, creamy frozen dessert. Simply peel the banana (insert a popsicle stick into the end if you like) and freeze it on a tray. Once frozen, wrap it in plastic.

Meal-Planning

There are three rules of thumb for creating the most powerful slimming meals possible:

* Use foods that are high in complex carbs.
* Avoid animal products.
* Eliminate oils or keep them to a bare minimum.

To make this very practical--and downright easy--I like to use a concept called the New Four Food Groups: vegetables, grains, legumes, and fruits. Together, they provide balanced nutrition and a maximal negative calorie effect. As you plan your meal, here is the best way to go about it.

1. Start with vegetables, usually including two different ones at each meal. Try broccoli, spinach, carrots, cauliflower, green beans, lima beans, Brussels sprouts, kale, asparagus, succotash, or any other. A sprinkle of lemon or lime juice can make green vegetables delectable. Or, if you like, add minced garlic, onion, or parsley. Steer clear of butter or margarine, sour cream, and other fatty toppings. Frozen vegetables are fine, but choose plain varieties, not those in cream sauce.

2. Second, add a generous amount of rice, pasta, potatoes, or any other grain or starchy food. Rice is one of the best for slimming down. It is extremely low in fat and calories, and very nutritious. At the grocery store, notice the variety of boxed rice dishes: curried rice, long grain and wild rice, brown rice, pecan rice, Basmati rice, risotto with tomato, or rice pilaf. But read the ingredients, as some contain chicken or beef fat. Nearby, you will see fabulous mixes for couscous, tabouli, and vegetarian burgers. Avoid any mixes with meat products or a high fat content. At the health food store, you will find organic short-grain rice, which is an excellent choice. See my special way of making brown rice in the recipe section.

Speaking of grains, everyone loves pasta. Whole-grain varieties are best, because they retain their natural fiber, but regular spaghetti is fine. Top with a tomato sauce, and choose those lowest in fat. Most breads are fine. Whole-grain varieties are always best. Corn is a nutritious grain. Savor its taste without butter, margarine, or oil.

Although potatoes are vegetables, they are similar to grains in their nutritional content. They are great baked, mashed (instant is fine), steamed, or boiled. Avoid hash browns, potato chips, and french fries. If you like, add a dab of Dijon mustard, ketchup, or soy sauce. Do not add milk to mashed potatoes, and use no butter, sour cream, margarine, cheese, or other fatty toppings. You may be amazed at the discovery (or rediscovery) of potato taste, especially if you pick a good organically produced baking potato and use a conventional oven.

3. After you have piled on the vegetables and grains, add a bean (legume) dish in smaller quantities. Vegetarian baked beans are available at most grocery stores and are very low in fat, loaded with complex carbs, and very convenient. Most groceries stock delicious, low-fat lentil soups. Health-food stores carry low-sodium varieties. Bean chili can be a hearty, low-fat meal. See the recipe section.

Be sure to try black beans, a Latin American favorite. They are extremely low in fat, packed with fiber, and delicious. Top with mild salsa or mustard. If you are new to black beans, buy them canned, rather than cooking up dried beans, which requires a lot more time. In case you were worrying, black beans do not seem to cause much gassiness.

Also in the legume category are soybean products. Marinated tempeh burgers are found at any health food store, along with various mixes to which tofu is added to make dozens of delicious main dishes, including, incredibly, a "scrambled eggless" breakfast. Their taste is a bit mellower than meat, but even dyed-in-the-wool steak eaters enjoy the flavor and texture of marinated tempeh, and most soon become ardent converts. Keep portions of tofu or tempeh modest. While they are lower in fat than many foods they replace, they are not nearly as low as other beans and bean products.

4. Fruits. Pears, oranges, cherries, strawberries, peaches, apples, bananas, pineapples, and just about anything other variety make great snacks, desserts, or garnishes for other foods. Try them fresh, frozen, chopped, in salads, or blended into fruit smoothies (see the recipe section.)

Modifying Recipes

Don't be afraid to modify recipes. Here are some hints that will help you take the fat out of old favorites.

* The amounts of oil added to recipes are often quite arbitrary. You can usually use much less, or even none at all. You may have to compensate with a little extra liquid to achieve the desired consistency. Once you have "reset" your taste for fat, you will automatically want to leave the grease out of the foods you prepare.

* Applesauce, mashed banana, prune purée, or canned pumpkin may be substituted for the fat or shortening in many baked goods.

* Health food stores sell Egg Replacer that does exactly that, drastically cutting down the fat content of baked goods. An egg-sized bit of mashed banana, applesauce, or tofu will also accomplish much the same thing in a baking recipe.

* TVP (textured vegetable protein), a de-fatted soy product sold at health food stores, replaces ground beef so well that some pizza companies and other ground beef users have already made the switch.

* Make soup thick and creamy by adding a potato. For soups that will be puréed, simply cook and purée the potato along with the other soup ingredients. For other soups, add instant mashed potato flakes or a cooked puréed potato.

* To make a stew "beefy," add a tablespoon of Tartex, Marmite, or Vegemite (flavorful yeast extracts sold in health food stores) per quart.

* Prepare pies with a single crust to reduce fat and calories (about 100 fewer calories per serving).

* Crumb crusts can be prepared with less fat than traditional flour-based crusts.

Cutting the Fat

Here are a few more tips to really cut the fat in your meals:

* Many baked goods, such as bagels, pretzels, and most breads, are usually low in fat, but check the labels. On the other hand, croissants, cakes, pies, and cookies are usually just the opposite. On labels, ingredients are listed in decreasing order of their quantities, so if oil is one of the first ingredients, there is probably more of it than if it is at the end of the list. Labels may note the actual fat content. It is often listed as "calories from fat" which you can divide by the total number of calories in the product to see the percentage of calories from fat. Ideally, it should be in the 10-15 percent range or below.

* Use a microwave oven to reheat foods that would otherwise stick to the pan.

* Watch out for avocados, olives, seeds, nuts, and nut products, which are among the very few plant products that are high in fat.

* Replace ice cream with fruit sorbet or a frozen fruit smoothie (see recipe section.)

* Travel is often a time of challenges for those trying to eat in a healthful way, but many fast-food restaurants have responded to the demand with baked potatoes and salad bars. Taco restaurants feature bean burritos (hold the cheese). In your car, bring along some fresh fruit or sandwiches. When you book a flight, request a pure vegetarian meal or a fruit plate; all airlines have them.

* Parties can be a challenge, too. When I am invited to a dinner party, I always say something along the lines of "I am trying to stick to vegetarian foods right now, and I don't want to put you to any trouble. How about if I bring along something, maybe a meatless spaghetti sauce?" Invariably, the host de-

clines my offer saying her husband is trying to bring down a high cholesterol level or her son is a vegetarian. Whatever he or she might really have been thinking, you have provided a good dinner suggestion far enough in advance to avert any problem. This is always better than politely eating little bits of what is served and having your host find out later that you were trying to eat healthy to lose weight. In case your host actually takes you up on the offer to bring food, you will find plenty of easy recipes in this book.

Fear of Frying?

Here are some tips on how to take the fat out of frying.

* For fat-free frying, the new non-stick pans work remarkably well.

* Instead of sautéing in oil, try this helpful tip: Put a quarter- to a half-cup of water in a saucepan on medium-high heat, and "sauté" onions, garlic, or other vegetables in simmering water. This usually takes about five minutes. Stir frequently, and add a little extra water if the vegetables begin to stick. You get a pleasant, lighter taste and skip the 240 calories that hide in two tablespoons of oil. This technique is called braising, and it works just as well with vegetable stock, wine, or dry sherry.

* When a recipe just won't work without sautéing or frying in oil, non-stick vegetable oil sprays allow you to do so with a fraction of the fat.

* Grilling and oven-roasting are great substitutes for frying. Try Oven Fries (see recipe section) instead of those deadly deep-fried french fries. At the store, look for baked versions of fried foods, like baked tortilla chips or potato chips.

Undressing Your Salad

It is easy to cut down on the oil in salad dressings, which is a good idea, because ordinary brands are packed with it. A salad made of one cup of romaine lettuce with half a tomato holds only 20 calories. But a tablespoon of Good Seasons Zesty Italian adds more than 9 grams of fat and 85 calories. A fifty-fifty mix of vinegar and oil adds about 8 grams of fat and 72 calories. A salad with just about any regular dressing has four to five times the calories of a salad without it.

* Check the low-fat or no-fat brands now available at the grocery store, often in the "dietetic section." Seasoned rice vinegar and balsamic vinegar also make great fat-free salad dressings, or try the recipes in the back of this book. Or do what I do, and sprinkle a little lemon or lime juice on salad or vegetables. A tablespoon of lemon or lime juice has no fat and only four calories. You may also find that you enjoy the taste of fresh spinach, chick peas, tomatoes, or other salad ingredients with no dressing at all.

* Replace the oil called for in salad dressing recipes with seasoned rice vinegar, vegetable stock, bean cooking liquid, or water.

* For a thicker dressing, use a cornstarch and water mixture as follows: Whisk one tablespoon of cornstarch with one cup of water. Heat in a small saucepan, stirring constantly, until thick and clear. Refrigerate. Use in place of oil in any salad dressing recipe. It will keep refrigerated for up to three weeks.

6

POWER DINNERS

Y ou have learned how foods can encourage a steady weight loss, which is accelerated by regular physical activity. If your body fat were a huge bag of water, you just poked a small hole in it. Slowly and surely it will start to drain out. In this section we will go a bit further.

TUNE UP YOUR MENU

* Use more whole, unmilled grains, like brown rice, rolled oats, and corn. They seem to release a bit fewer of their calories, compared to pasta or bread, where the grain has been pulverized and, in some cases, the fiber has been removed. Let them play a greater role in your diet. If you have not tried my way of cooking brown rice, please do. It can give a terrific boost to your menu.

* Give vegetables a more prominent role in your menu, too. Serve steamed spinach, Swiss chard, cauliflower, or broccoli florets with a touch of lemon juice as a salad or appetizer, in addition to vegetables with your main dish.

* Think raw. Many people report remarkable weight reductions when they include more raw fruits and vegetables in their diets. This is partly because these foods are extremely low in fat and high in fiber and carbohydrate, but there may be other reasons that science has not yet unraveled. People with even stubborn weight problems have benefited greatly by including more raw vegetables and fruits.

* When you select raw vegetables, don't rely on iceberg lettuce; it's mostly water. For a salad, try fresh spinach and the other delightful greens in the produce department. Add peppers, celery, carrots, and cauliflower, and throw in some cooked

chickpeas or whatever else you might like. Happily, it is now easier to find vegetables produced without pesticides. Skip dressings that include oil. You might want to enjoy the taste of vegetables without added flavorings.

* Think about the timing of your dinners. If an overly full daytime schedule pushes your dinner later and later, you may find yourself more likely to compromise your menu or even to binge. In that case, try to eat earlier, even if you return to work or other chores afterward. On the other hand, if you tend to eat so early that you end up hungry before bedtime, be sure to have some good healthy nibbles on hand for bedtime snacks.

CHOOSING A POWER MENU

The recipes in this book are low in fat and high in complex carbs. However, some are particularly remarkable. The following items, all of which are found in the recipe section, draw <u>less than five percent</u> of their calories from fat. From this menu, you can plan your power dinners for maximal weight loss.

SOUPS AND STEWS

Lentil Barley Soup
Simply Wonderful Vegetable Stew
Split Pea Soup
Garden Vegetable Soup
Curried Lentil Soup
Autumn Stew
Potato and Cabbage Soup
Black Bean Soup

SALADS

Serve with Fat-free Dressing, Piquant Dressing, Balsamic Vinaigrette, Curry Dressing, any commercially available non-fat dressing, or lemon or lime juice.

Mixed Greens Salad
Four Bean Salad
Quick and Colorful Couscous Salad
Red Potato Salad
Spinach Salad with Curry Dressing
Aztec Salad
Pasta Salad
White Bean Salad
Cucumber Salad

MAIN DISHES AND QUICK MEALS

Very Primo Pasta
Super Chili
Quick Chili
Shepherd's Pie
Crostini with Sun-Dried Tomatoes
Bean Weenies

For convenience, you can also use any variety of canned beans, such as vegetarian baked beans or black beans.

VEGETABLES

Broccoli with Fat-free Dressing
Braised Cabbage
Green Beans with Sweet Onions
Roasted Yams
Oven Fries
Golden Potatoes

GRAINS

Brown Rice
Quick Confetti Rice
Bulgur
Spanish Bulgur
Couscous
Polenta

DESSERTS

Cranberry Apple Crisp
Tropical Delight
Pumpkin Raisin Cookies
Prune Whip
Baked Apples
Poached Pears

BEST RESTAURANT CHOICES

When choosing restaurants, the best choices are Japanese, Chinese, and other Asian cuisines, Mexican, Italian, Middle-eastern, and Indian. Here are some common menu items you might look for:

Japanese- Start with miso soup, a delicious Japanese tradition. Follow it with vegetable sushi, in which sliced cucumber, radish, spinach, carrots, or other vegetables are combined with seasoned rice and wrapped in toasted nori, a nutritious sea vegetable, and served with delightful condiments. Avoid fish or shellfish sushi of any variety. Have some sides of spinach, watercress, or other vegetables.

Chinese- The menu will vary dramatically, depending on the part of China its cuisine reflects. Szechuan and Hunan restaurant have particularly savory dishes. The menu is usually divided into meat, poultry, fish, and vegetable dishes. The vegetables are, by far, the healthiest and most interesting. They are not just a couple of green beans on a plate. They are main dishes in exotic sauces, designed to be served on a generous bed of rice. Try the garlic broccoli, eggplant, or spinach. They will also have several bean curd (tofu) dishes, some of which are deep fried and dripping with grease, while others are cooked more sensibly and mixed with vegetables in a spicy brown sauce. Empty the accompanying bowl of rice onto your plate and top it with a smaller portion of your vegetable dish, which always arrives in portions big enough to feed an army. Although traditional Chinese cuisine is among the lowest in fat of any in the world, the Westernized restaurant versions are often greased up in anticipation of local tastes. Because each dish is made to order, it is no problem for the chef to minimize the use of cooking oils, if you ask.

Mexican- Have a bean burrito (hold the cheese) with rice and salad. If you're feeling adventurous, they'll be glad to add some jalapeno peppers. At other Latin American restaurants, beans, salsa, rice, tortillas, and salads are a wonderful feast.

Italian- Try minestrone or pasta e fagioli, a delicious pasta and bean soup, perhaps with appetizers of asparagus or artichoke, or a mixed green salad, followed by linguine or other pasta with a tomato/basil sauce and sides of spinach or the deep green, leafy broccoli-rab. The only risk is whether the restaurateur is in-clined to put olive oil in everything, as some are. Ask them to go easy on it or leave it out.

Middle-Eastern- Try the couscous, tabouli, spinach pies, and hummus with flat breads.

Indian- Indian restaurants turn the humblest foods into culinary masterpieces. Spinach, potatoes, lentils, chickpeas, and endless other vegetables are artistically spiced and served with rice and fresh breads that put Western breads to shame. The Achilles' heel of Indian cuisine is the overly generous use of <u>gee</u>, a clarified butter that will expand your girth as surely as the unclarified varieties. The rice dishes and breads are the healthiest offerings.

French- There is nothing like French vegetables: carefully se-lected, exquisitely prepared, and elegantly presented. Ask that they be steamed and that sauces stay in the kitchen; a little lemon or vinegar will allow you to savour the taste of vegeta-bles as they should be.

American- The country that practically invented the heart at-tack is not entirely a culinary wasteland. Drawing on its immi-grant roots, American restaurants often have spaghetti with to-mato sauce, whether or not it appears on the menu. More and more restaurants offer veggie burgers. They also have baked potatoes and will gladly make up a vegetable plate. While newcomers to healthy eating might consider vegetable plates to be just a combination of side dishes, they will soon find them to be more like palettes of nature's artistry, designed to complement your own. The U.S. National Restaurant Association asked all its members in 1991 to feature vegetarian dishes, because, at that time, about one in five diners looked for them. If you don't see them on the menu, by all means ask. And don't be afraid to ask for modifications of menu items.

If you have Ethiopian, Greek, or Caribbean restaurants near you, you will find more treats to explore (along with some menu items you will want to avoid.) Enjoy the world of healthful eating.

In the Fast-Food Lane

Fast-food restaurants carry dozens of artery-clogging, waistline-padding, and downright dangerous products. But they also have offerings that are healthy. Shopping mall food courts, in particular, have a growing selection of specialty fast-food outlets featuring Chinese, Japanese, Mexican, and Italian cuisine. I recently had a lovely pasta primavera topped with sliced broccoli, carrots, and other delicious vegetables and tomato sauce on the side, offered with a huge green salad, garlic bread, and sparkling water, all served up in less than two minutes--fast-food, Italian-style! Here are some items to look for at fast-food restaurants:

* Burger restaurants: Look for salad bars, featuring pasta salads, chick peas, bean dishes, fresh fruit, apple sauce, and fresh greens. Try the baked potatoes with vegetable toppings, minus any fatty condiments. Some chains have baked or refried beans, and some are even experimenting with vegetarian burgers, which may or may not be low in fat.

* Fried chicken outlets often feature corn on the cob, various kinds of rice, mashed potatoes, baked beans, and salads. The chicken itself is never truly low in fat, no matter how it is prepared.

* Mexican fast-food restaurants offer bean burritos (hold the

cheese), Spanish rice, and salads.

* Submarine sandwich shops: Have a veggie sub and a nice big salad.

TROUBLE-SHOOTING

Your results may be speedy, but if they come slowly, be patient. Slow weight loss is more likely to be permanent than very rapid weight loss. But if you have tried this program and have not lost weight at all, then let's review the basics: Are you still using any oily foods, such as salad dressings, peanut butter, or margarine? Were there any animal products in your foods? Remember, even chicken and fish are nowhere near fat-free, and because they have no complex carbs at all, they do nothing to speed up your metabolism. Is alcohol contributing to your weight? If you had problems in any of these areas, now is the time to address them squarely. There are always solutions, and tremendous rewards waiting for you.

Are you having trouble sticking to healthy foods when you are with friends? It may be that you are concerned that they will not sympathize with your new and healthful way of eating or will give you a hard time. If so, I have noticed a remarkable thing in the past few years. Every time the subject of foods comes up in conversation, health concerns inevitably follow. People know very well by now that fat and cholesterol are risky business, and they know that the old-fashioned approach to diets is essentially futile over the long run. Many people are becoming vegetarians or near-vegetarians, or at least recognize that they should be. So stop worrying. Ask for their support. You've only got one body. You would not put the wrong fuel in your car just because others did so. Why put the wrong fuel in your body?

Are you getting enough sleep? Chronically tired people are often tempted to prop up their flagging spirits with food, often the most fattening ones, and they rarely have enough energy to exercise. A good night's sleep can do you a world of good.

Some people have digestive troubles. Any major change in

your diet can be a temporary challenge. A meat-eater who becomes a vegetarian suddenly has to adapt to a high-fiber diet and may have a little indigestion or gas. If a vegetarian were to become a meat-eater, a similar problem could occur. If this happens to you, try to pin down which is the problem food. Pinto or garbanzo beans, for example, may be a problem, while black beans are not. Also, have more grains, such as rice, and have smaller amounts of beans. For some people, the problem food may be broccoli or cabbage. Give yourself a break from that food, and come back to it later. Our digestive tracts often adjust over time.

This program is elegantly simple, yet is the most effective way to control your weight permanently. The great part is that there is no need to count calories, skip meals, or eat small portions. You can let your taste buds and your appetite enjoy a wide range of foods, and enjoy them in a slimmer, healthier body.

7

OPTIONAL, BUT POWERFUL, PHYSICAL ACTIVITY

Modern civilization has made most of us far too sedentary. We have eliminated much of the walking, running, or other physical activities that kept our ancestors fit and got our blood moving when we were younger. You do not have to exercise to take advantage of the negative calorie effect, because foods themselves can increase your metabolism and help you lose weight whether you exercise or not. But it is terrific to "get physical" on a regular basis, for four reasons:

First, movement burns calories: Every movement you make, whether it is blinking your eyes or lifting a grand piano, burns some calories. The more you move, the more calories you burn.

Second, regular physical activity boosts your metabolism. Calories are burned more quickly, not only while you are exercising, but also afterward for a period of time.

Third, any kind of exercise helps preserve your muscles. Muscle tissue is much better than fat tissue at burning off calories. If your muscles waste away from inactivity, your body burns calories slower.

Fourth, physical activity helps regulate the appetite. Twenty minutes of exercise before dinner slightly reduces the tendency to overeat. This seems to be particularly true for activities that warm the body, such as tennis, running, or dancing. Some people experience an <u>increase</u> in appetite after cooling exercises, such as swimming. Unfortunately, it is likely that overweight people experience less (or even none) of the exercise-induced change in appetite than do normal-weight individuals, so this may be a mechanism that helps you <u>stay</u> thin rather than helping you to get there.[37]

There are many other benefits of physical activity, from reduced risk of heart disease and cancer to more energy and a more relaxed outlook on life. You may find that you will sleep more soundly when your body is tired from exercise. In turn, better sleep makes you feel like taking care of yourself.

HOW MUCH ACTIVITY?

You can get the benefits of physical activity without pumping iron or jogging for miles at the crack of dawn. My recommendation is simply a half-hour walk every day, or, if you prefer, an hour three times per week. This sounds very modest, but it is more than enough to do the job.

Pick a place to walk that is enjoyable for you. Enjoy the sights, sounds, and smells. Feel free to substitute any equivalent activity instead of walking. Here are some examples, with the number of calories they burn for a 150-pound adult. For a 100-pound person, subtract one-third. For a 200-pound person, add one-third.

CALORIE-BURNING EXAMPLES

A brisk half-hour walk	220
A leisurely half-hour bicycle ride	120
A half-hour bicycle ride at moderate speed	200
A half-hour leisurely swim	140
A half-hour fast swim	250
A slow haif-hour jog	370
A quick half-hour jog	460
Running in place for half an hour	325
A half-hour of singles tennis	200
A half-hour of cross-country skiing	350
Jumping rope for half an hour	375

The key is to have fun, because if it's fun, you'll stick with it, and it is much more important that activities be regular than that they be vigorous. If you like dancing, gardening, bike-riding, a run with your dog, or a vigorous walk in the woods, then off you go! Vary your activities to keep them interesting. Get a friend or neighbor to join you if you can. Making it a scheduled social event decreases the possibility of your drifting back into sedentary living.

At work, use the stairs instead of the elevator. If you have access to a health club, you will find all sorts of ways to turn exercise into pleasure. The old gym has really been transformed into a place that is tailored to individual needs.

Do not overdo it. Lots of people start an exercise program much too aggressively and soon become weary of it or feel defeated by it. So let's not even use the word "exercise." The point is to enjoy the use of your body so you will want to keep it up. Start slow, particularly if you have been sedentary for some time. If you are over 40 or have any history of illness or joint problems, talk over your plans with your doctor.

Take a moment now, and think about your schedule. When is a time that you can reliably break free? Evening? Early morning? Late afternoon? Which is better for you--daily or three times per week? Is there another activity you would like to substitute some or all of the time? Would you like to join a club? And is there someone you can take with you?

If you have been on a low-calorie diet, you should switch to a low-fat, high-carb menu with no calorie restriction before you begin any program of regular vigorous exercise. The reason is that the low-calorie diet has probably slowed down your metabolism. Even though exercise will boost the metabolic rate of most people, it can actually have the opposite effect on people who have been starving themselves. So stop the calorie limit first. Then, after a couple of weeks, add physical activity.

Afterword

In this book, we have focused on the science of weight control. But there is so much more that you may want to learn about. Along with other lifestyle changes, foods can actually help reverse heart disease, prevent many cases of cancer and improve cancer survival, yield dramatic improvements in diabetes and high blood pressure, and help with many other conditions from appendicitis to varicose veins. These are covered in detail in my other books, which are listed in the front of this volume. I hope you will take a look at them and try their recipes as well.

Let me wish you the very best of success with your new venture. Please share this book with other people, and let me know how it works for you.

MENUS

*Items which are capitalized
are included in the recipe section.*

DAY ONE

Breakfast

slice of fresh melon
Buckwheat Corncakes, page 100
maple syrup or unsweetened fruit preserves

Lunch

Lentil Barley Soup, page 115
Mixed Greens Salad, page 130
with Balsamic Vinaigrette, page 129
whole wheat roll

Dinner

Pasta with Roasted Summer Vegetables, page 154
White Bean Salad, page 136
Steamed Kale, page 142
Poached Pears, page 184

DAY TWO

Breakfast

1/2 grapefruit
Creamy Oatmeal, page 101
with raisins and cinnamonslice of whole
grain toast with unsweetened fruit preserves

Lunch

Missing Egg Sandwich, page 166
Red Potato Salad, page 132
fresh fruit

Dinner

Quick Chili, page 157
Brown Rice, page 148
Terrific Tacos, page 168
Mixed Greens Salad, page 130
with Piquant Dressing, page 128
Tropical Delight, page 177

Day Three

Breakfast

Oatmeal Waffles, page 99
strawberries and bananas or
unsweetened fruit preserves
Apricot Smoothie, page 106

Lunch

Potato and Cabbage Soup, page 124
Four Bean Salad, page 130
Pumpkin Spice Muffin, page 108

Dinner

Pita Pizzas, page 170
Pasta Salad, page 135
Broccoli with Fat-free Dressing, page 140
Quick Rice Pudding, page 178

DAY FOUR

Breakfast

melon wedge
Breakfast Bulgur, page 101
Stewed Prunes, page 104

Lunch

Creamy Lima Soup, page 121
Quick and Colorful Couscous Salad, page 131
Quick Confetti Rice, page 148
rye bread
Pumpkin Raisin Cookies, page 181

Dinner

Shepherd's Pie, page 161
Spinach Salad with Curry Dressing, page 133
Braised Cabbage, page 140
Quick and Easy Brown Bread, page 110

DAY FIVE

Breakfast

Scrambled Tofu, page 102
Braised Potatoes, page 103
Applesauce, page 104

Lunch

Split Pea Soup, page 117
Red Potato Salad, page 132
whole grain bread or roll
Baked Apples, page 183

Dinner

Autumn Stew, page 123
Brown Rice, page 148
Steamed Kale, page 142
Quick and Easy Brown Bread, page 110
Berry Cobbler, page 176

DAY SIX

Breakfast

cold cereal with soymilk or rice milk
whole grain toast
Strawberry Smoothie, page 105

Lunch

Aztec Salad, page 134
Cornbread, page 111
Simply Wonderful Winter Squash, page 141

Dinner

Lasagne, page 163
Mixed Greens Salad, page 130
with Fat-free Dressing, page 128
Broccoli with Fat-free Dressing, page 140
Garlic Bread, page 112
Prune Whip, page 182

DAY SEVEN

Breakfast

Double Bran Muffin, page 108
hot cereal with soymilk or rice milk
fresh fruit

Lunch

Curried Lentil Soup, page 120
Mixed Greens Salad, page 130
with Curry Dressing, page 129
Golden Potatoes, page 145
Gingerbread, page 181

Dinner

Spinach and Mushroom Fritatta, page 162
Pasta Salad, page 135
Broccoli with Fat-free Dressing, page 140
Crostini with Sun Dried Tomatoes, page 171
Bread Pudding, page 179

A Few Ingredients That May Be New to You

Most of the ingredients in the recipes are common and widely available in grocery stores. A few which may be unfamiliar are described below.

Balsamic vinegar--A delightful and mellow-flavored wine vinegar, available in most grocery stores.

Low-sodium baking powder--Made without sodium bicarbonate, and available in natural food stores.

Lite soy sauce--Less sodium than regular brands. Compare labels to get the brand that is lowest.

Reduced-fat tofu--The world's most adaptable ingredient in a lower fat form. Silken tofu is a smooth, delicate variety that is excellent for sauces, cream soups, and dips, and can be stored without refrigeration for up to a year. Refrigerate after opening. One popular brand, Mori-Nu, is available in most grocery stores.

Rice milk--A mild-flavored beverage made from rice, which avoids the lactose, animal protein, animal fat, and contaminants in cow's milk. Use in place of dairy milk on cereal and in most recipes. Rice Dream and Eden Rice are two brands available in natural food stores and some supermarkets.

Roasted red peppers--To add great flavor and color to a variety of dishes, roast your own or purchase them already roasted, packed in water, in most grocery stores.

Seasoned rice vinegar--A mild-flavored vinegar, seasoned with sugar and salt. Great for salad dressings and on cooked vegetables. Available in most grocery stores.

Soymilk--A milk-like beverage made from soybeans, available in a variety of flavors, as well as in low-fat and vitamin- and calcium-fortified versions. See which flavors you like best. Available in natural food stores and in many supermarkets.

Textured vegetable protein (TVP)--Made from defatted soy flour, TVP has a meaty texture when rehydrated with boiling water. Easy to use and an excellent meat substitute in sauces, chilis, and stews. Available in natural food stores.

Whole wheat pastry flour--Milled from soft spring wheat, it retains the bran and germ and, at the same time, produces lighter-textured baked goods than regular whole wheat flour. Available in natural food stores.

BREAKFASTS

Start your day out right with a good breakfast. Wholegrain cereals, breads, baked goods, pancakes, and waffles make excellent breakfast fare. Add a bit of fresh fruit, and you have a meal to keep you going all morning long.

Whole Wheat Pancakes

Four simple ingredients are all it takes to make nutritious, satisfying pancakes. Serve them with natural fruit preserves or maple syrup.

1	cup whole wheat pastry flour or whole wheat flour
2	teaspoons low-sodium baking powder
$1^1/_3$	cups soymilk or rice milk
1	tablespoon maple syrup

Stir flour and baking powder together. Add the milk and syrup and stir enough to remove the lumps, but do not overmix. Pour small amounts of batter onto a preheated nonstick griddle or skillet which has been lightly oil-sprayed. Cook until the tops bubble. Turn with a spatula and cook the second side until golden brown. Serve immediately.

Makes 16 3-inch pancakes

Nutrition information per pancake:
37 calories (7% from fat); 1 g protein; 7 g carbohydrate; 0.3 g fat; 62 mg sodium; 44 mg calcium

Oatmeal Waffles

Oatmeal waffles are substantial and slightly moist, a bit like eating oatmeal with a crunchy crust. They are easy to prepare and contain no added fat.

2	cups rolled oats
2	cups water
1	banana
1	tablespoon maple syrup
¼	teaspoon salt
1	teaspoon vanilla

Place all ingredients into a blender and blend until smooth. Pour into a preheated, oil-sprayed waffle iron. Cook for 10 minutes without lifting the lid. Serve with fresh fruit.

Note: The batter should be easily pourable. If it becomes thickened with standing, add a bit more water to achieve desired consistency.

Makes 4 waffles

Nutrition information per waffle:
203 calories (14% from fat); 8 g protein; 33 g carbohydrate; 3 g fat; 134 mg sodium; 26 mg calcium

Buckwheat Corncakes

Buckwheat adds a wonderful, hearty flavor to these easily prepared pancakes. I like to serve them with homemade applesauce and one of the vegetarian sausages available in most natural food stores.

½	cup buckwheat flour
½	cup cornmeal
½	teaspoon low-sodium baking powder
¼	teaspoon baking soda
½	ripe banana, mashed
1½	tablespoons brown sugar
1	tablespoon vinegar
1-1¼	cups soymilk or rice milk

Stir flour, cornmeal, baking powder, and baking soda together in a mixing bowl. In a separate bowl, combine mashed banana, sugar, vinegar and 2 cups of soymilk or rice milk. Pour liquid ingredients into the flour mixture and stir just enough to remove lumps and make a pourable batter. Add a bit more milk if the mixture seems too thick.

Preheat a nonstick skillet or griddle. Spray lightly with a nonstick spray. Pour small amounts of batter onto the heated surface and cook until the tops bubble. Turn with a spatula and cook the second side until golden brown. Serve immediately with maple syrup and fruit preserves.

Makes 16 3-inch pancakes

Nutrition information per pancake:
80 calories (5% from fat); 2 g protein; 17 g carbohydrate; 0.5 g fat; 38 mg sodium; 16 mg calcium

Creamy Oatmeal

Once you've tried this delicious, creamy oatmeal, you'll never want it any other way. It's made with Rice Dream, a delicious rice milk sold in natural food stores and many supermarkets.

1	cup rolled oats
3	cups vanilla Rice Dream

Combine rolled oats and Rice Dream in a saucepan over medium heat. Bring to a simmer and cook 1 minute. Cover the pan, turn off the heat and let stand 3 minutes. Serves 2

Nutrition information per serving:
290 calories (17% from fat); 12 g protein; 50 g carbohydrate; 5 g fat; 136 mg sodium; 83 mg calcium

Breakfast Bulgur

Bulgur wheat makes a quick hot breakfast cereal. It has a wonderful crunchy texture and nutty flavor.

2	cups water
1	cup bulgur wheat
¼	teaspoon cinnamon
¼	teaspoon salt
¼	cup raisins
1	cup soymilk or rice milk

Bring water to boil in a saucepan then add the bulgur, cinnamon, salt, and raisins. Cover and simmer over low heat 10 minutes. Add the soymilk or rice milk, cover and simmer another 5 minutes. Serve with soymilk or rice milk and maple syrup if desired. Serves 3 to 4

Nutrition information per serving:
163 calories (4% from fat); 6 g protein; 34 g carbohydrate; 1 g fat; 160 mg sodium; 42 mg calcium

Scrambled Tofu

Scrambled tofu tastes remarkably like scrambled eggs, without the saturated fat or cholesterol. The recipe which follows can be embellished with additional vegetables, such as sliced mushrooms and celery, diced zucchini, or grated carrot. Cook these with the onions. Serve with toasted English muffins, Braised Potatoes, and apple chutney. For convenience, you may wish to try boxed tofu scrambler mix, available at health food stores.

½	cup water
3	teaspoons lite soy sauce
½	medium onion, chopped
2	cups sliced mushrooms
1	pound firm tofu, diced or crumbled
1-½	teaspoons curry powder

Heat the water and soy sauce in a large nonstick skillet and cook the onion and mushrooms for 5 minutes. Add the tofu, then stir in the curry powder. Continue cooking 3 to 4 minutes.

Serves 4

Nutrition information per serving:
114 calories (24% from fat); 13 g protein; 8 g carbohydrate; 3 g fat; 158 mg sodium; 156 mg calcium

Braised Potatoes

These quick potatoes are delicious with ketchup, barbecue sauce, or with black bean chili and spicy salsa. Be sure to use a nonstick skillet.

4	large red or gold potatoes
4	teaspoons lite soy sauce
½	cup water
1	onion, chopped
1	teaspoon chili powder
	black pepper (optional)

Scrub the potatoes, but do not peel them. Cut them into ¼-inch thick slices and steam over boiling water until just tender when pierced with a sharp knife.

In a large nonstick skillet, braise the onion in water and 2 teaspoons of soy sauce until soft, about 3 minutes. Add the potatoes, chili powder, and remaining soy sauce and stir gently to mix. Cook over medium heat, stirring occasionally, for 3 to 5 minutes. Sprinkle with fresh ground black pepper if desired.

Serves 2 to 4

Nutrition information per serving:
200 calories (1% from fat); 6 g protein; 43 g carbohydrate; 0.3 g fat; 215 mg sodium; 34 mg calcium

Applesauce

Applesauce is delicious on toast, pancakes, and hot cereal. For a simple dessert, sprinkle it with fat-free granola.

6	large green apples
½-1	cup undiluted apple juice concentrate
½	teaspoon cinnamon

Peel the apples if desired, then core and dice them into a large pan. Add apple juice concentrate to just cover bottom of pan, then cook over low heat until apples are soft. Mash slightly with a fork if desired, then stir in cinnamon. Serve hot or cold.

Serves 8

Nutrition information per serving:
124 calories (3% from fat); 0.5 g protein; 30 g carbohydrate; 0.4 g fat; 0 mg sodium; 6 mg calcium

Stewed Prunes

Prunes are a delicious source of vitamins, minerals, and fiber. Serve them for breakfast with soymilk or rice milk, or use them to make Prune Whip on page 182.

    1   cup dried prunes
    1   cup water

Combine prunes and water in a covered saucepan and simmer for 20 minutes, until prunes are tender. Serve hot or cold.

Serves 3 to 4

Nutrition information per serving:
113 calories (1% from fat); 1 g protein; 27 g carbohydrate; 0.1 g fat; 2 mg sodium; 24 mg calcium

Smoothies

Although smoothies have been included in the breakfast section, they also make wonderful desserts. The secret to making a good smoothie is using frozen fruit, to make it really thick and cold. Try the following smoothies for starters, then begin experimenting with your own combinations.

Strawberry Smoothie

Try this cold, thick smoothie with whole grain cereal or muffins for a delicious and satisfying breakfast. You can buy frozen strawberries or freeze your own in an airtight container. To freeze bananas, peel them and break into inch-long pieces. Pack loosely in an airtight container and freeze. Bananas will keep in the freezer for about two months, strawberries for six months.

1	cup frozen strawberries
1	large frozen banana, cut into 1-inch pieces
½-1	cup unsweetened apple juice

Place all ingredients into blender and process on high speed until smooth. You may have to stop the blender occasionally and move the unblended fruit to the center with a spatula in order to get the smoothie smooth!

Serves 2

Nutrition information per serving:
97 calories (3% from fat); 1 g protein; 22 g carbohydrate; 0.3 g fat; 5 mg sodium; 17 mg calcium

Peach Sunrise

1	peach, sliced and frozen
¾-1	cup soymilk (vanilla or plain)
1	teaspoon sugar (optional)

Combine all ingredients in a blender and process until smooth. Serve immediately.

Serves 1

Nutrition information per serving:
156 calories (9% from fat); 4 g protein; 29 g carbohydrate; 1.5 g fat; 68 mg sodium; 77 mg calcium

Apricot Smoothie

1	cup frozen banana pieces
1	cup frozen apricots
¼	cup undiluted apple juice concentrate
¾	cup soymilk or rice milk

Combine all ingredients in a blender and process until smooth. Serve immediately.

Serves 2

Nutrition information per serving:
181 calories (6% from fat); 3 g protein; 40 g carbohydrate; 1 g fat; 44 mg sodium; 58 mg calcium

MUFFINS AND BREADS

Pumpkin Spice Muffins

2	cups whole wheat flour or whole wheat pastry flour
1	tablespoon low-sodium baking powder
½	teaspoon baking soda
½	teaspoon salt
½	teaspoon cinnamon
½	teaspoon nutmeg
1	cup sugar
1	15-ounce can solid-pack pumpkin
½	cup water
½	cup raisins

Preheat oven to 375°. Mix flour, baking powder, baking soda, salt, cinnamon, nutmeg, and sugar. Add the pumpkin, water, and raisins, and stir until just mixed. Lightly oil-spray muffin cups and fill to the top. Bake 25 to 30 minutes, until tops of muffins bounce back when pressed lightly. Remove from oven and let stand 1 to 2 minutes, then remove muffins from pan. When muffins are cool, store in an airtight container.

Makes 10 to 12 muffins

Nutrition information per muffin:
137 calories (0.4% from fat); 3 g protein; 31 g carbohydrate; 0.1 g fat; 128 mg sodium; 80 mg calcium

Double Bran Muffins

The secret to these wholesome, fruity muffins is prune puree, which makes them moist without added fat. Prune puree is marketed under the names WonderSlim and Lekvar, or you can even use a 4-ounce jar of prune baby food. The muffins will be quite moist when they first come out of the oven, so let them stand a few minutes before serving.

2   cups whole wheat flour or whole wheat pastry flour

¾   cup wheat bran

¾   cup oat bran

½   teaspoon salt

1   teaspoon baking soda

1   teaspoon cinnamon

¼   teaspoon nutmeg

1   apple, finely chopped or grated (use the food processor)

½   cup raisins

1-½   cups soymilk or rice milk

1-½   tablespoons vinegar

¼   cup prune puree or 1 4-ounce jar of baby prunes

1/3   cup molasses

Preheat oven to 350°. Mix the flour, brans, salt, soda and spices. In a separate bowl mix the remaining ingredients. Stir the wet ingredients into the flour mixture until mixed. Spoon into muffin pans which have been sprayed with a nonstick spray and bake until tops bounce back when lightly pressed, about 25 minutes. Let stand 1 to 2 minutes, then remove from pan and let stand an additional 5 to 10 minutes.

Makes 12 muffins

Nutrition information per muffin:
171 calories (5% from fat); 5 g protein; 35 g carbohydrate; 1 g fat; 199 mg sodium; 52 mg calcium

Applesauce Muffins

2	cups whole wheat pastry flour
1	tablespoon low-sodium baking powder
½	teaspoon baking soda
½	teaspoon salt
½	teaspoon cinnamon
½	cup sugar
1	15-ounce can applesauce
½	cup water
½	cup raisins

Preheat oven to 375°. Mix dry ingredients. Add the applesauce, water, and raisins. Stir until just mixed. Lightly spray muffin cups with nonstick spray and fill to the top. Bake 25 to 30 minutes, until tops of muffins bounce back when pressed lightly. Remove from oven and let stand 1 to 2 minutes, then remove muffins from pan. When muffins are cool, store in an airtight container.

Makes 10 to 12 muffins

Nutrition information per muffin:
140 calories (0% from fat); 3 g protein; 32 g carbohydrate; 0 g fat; 127 mg sodium; 71 mg calcium

Quick and Easy Brown Bread

This bread, reminiscent of good old Boston brown bread, is sweet and moist, without any added fat or oil. It can be mixed in a jiffy and requires no kneading or rising. It keeps well and makes wonderful toast.

1-½	cups lowfat soymilk
2	tablespoons vinegar
2	cups whole wheat flour
1	cup unbleached flour
2	teaspoons baking soda
½	teaspoon salt

½   cup molasses
½   cup raisins

Preheat oven to 325°. Mix soymilk with vinegar and set aside. In a large mixing bowl, stir dry ingredients together. Add molasses, soymilk-vinegar mixture, and raisins. Stir batter until thoroughly mixed, but do not overmix. Spoon batter into a nonstick or lightly oil-sprayed loaf pan and bake at 325° for one hour.

Makes 1 loaf: 20 slices

Nutrition information per slice:
111 calories (3% from fat); 3 g protein; 24 g carbohydrate; 0.4 g fat; 149 mg sodium; 42 mg calcium

Cornbread

This cornbread is quick and easy to prepare and contains no eggs, cholesterol, or added fat.

1-½   cups soymilk
1-½   tablespoons vinegar
1   cup cornmeal
1   cup flour (unbleached or whole wheat pastry)
2   teaspoons low-sodium baking powder
½   teaspoon baking soda
½   teaspoon salt

Preheat oven to 425°. Combine soymilk and vinegar and set aside. Stir dry ingredients together in a large bowl then add the soymilk mixture and mix until just blended. Spread evenly in a 9 x 9-inch baking dish which has been lightly sprayed with a nonstick spray, and bake for 25 to 30 minutes. Serve hot.

Serves 8

Nutrition information per serving:
124 calories (4% from fat); 3 g protein; 26 g carbohydrate; 0.6 g fat; 180 mg sodium; 65 mg calcium

Garlic Bread

1	head garlic
1	baguette or loaf of French bread, sliced
1-2	teaspoon Italian Seasoning

Roast the garlic by baking the whole, unpeeled head in a 400° oven (or toaster oven) until it feels soft when gently squeezed. This will take about 30 minutes. Peel the cloves, or squeeze them out of their skin, then mash them into a paste with a fork. Mix in the herbs if desired, then spread onto the sliced bread. Wrap tightly in foil and Bake at 350° for 20 minutes.

Serves 8

Nutrition information per serving:

91 calories (1% from fat); 3 g protein; 18.5 g carbohydrate; 0.1 g fat; 179 mg sodium; 12 mg calcium

SOUPS

Lentil Barley Soup

This soup is as easy to prepare as it is hearty and satisfying. Serve it with warm bread or muffins and a salad.

½	cup lentils, rinsed
¼	cup pearl barley
4	cups water or vegetable stock
1	small onion, chopped
1	carrot, diced
1	stalk celery, sliced
$^1/_8$	teaspoon oregano
$^1/_8$	teaspoon ground cumin
$^1/_8$	teaspoon red pepper flakes
$^1/_8$	teaspoon black pepper
¾	teaspoon salt

Place all ingredients except salt into a large pot and bring to a simmer. Cover and cook for 1 hour, stirring occasionally, until lentils and barley are tender. Add salt to taste.

Serves 8

Nutrition information per serving:
70 calories (1% from fat); 4 g protein; 14 g carbohydrate; 0.1 g fat; 200 mg sodium; 20 mg calcium

Vegetable Stew

This delicious stew contains relatively few ingredients and is quick to prepare. Serve it with a fresh green salad and crusty sourdough French bread.

1 ½	cups water
2	medium onions, chopped
2	cloves garlic, minced
1	28-ounce can chopped tomatoes, including liquid
1	large green bell pepper, seeded and diced
6	medium red potatoes, unpeeled, cut into 1-inch chunks
1	teaspoon basil
1	teaspoon oregano
1	teaspoon mixed Italian herbs
¼	teaspoon black pepper
¼	teaspoon salt
1-2	cups green peas, fresh or frozen

Heat ½ cup of water in a large pot and cook the onions and garlic until the onion is soft, about 5 minutes. Add the tomatoes, bell pepper, potatoes, remaining water and seasonings. Bring to a simmer, then cover and cook, stirring occasionally, until potatoes are just tender, about 20 minutes. Add extra water if necessary to prevent sticking. Stir in peas and continue cooking until heated through.

Serves 6 to 8

Nutrition information per serving:
156 calories (2% from fat); 5 g protein; 33 g carbohydrate; 0.3 g fat; 250 mg sodium; 53 mg calcium

Split Pea Soup

This simple one-pot soup contains no added fat, and is perfect for a cold, rainy day.

2	cups split peas, rinsed
6	cups water
1	medium onion, chopped
1	cup carrots, sliced or diced
1	cup celery, sliced
1	large potato, peeled and diced
2	cloves garlic, minced
½	teaspoon marjoram
½	teaspoon basil
¼	teaspoon ground cumin
¼	teaspoon black pepper
1	teaspoon salt
	pinch cayenne

Combine the split peas in a large pot with the remaining ingredients. Bring to a simmer, then cover loosely and cook until the peas are tender, 1 to 2 hours.

Serves 6 to 8

Nutrition information per serving:
158 calories (2% from fat); 9 g protein; 29 g carbohydrate; 0.4 g fat; 282 mg sodium; 30 mg calcium

Creamy Curried Carrot Soup

It's hard to believe that such a simple soup could be so delicious. This soup is a rich source of beta-carotene. Soy milk keeps it free of lactose and animal protein.

1	onion, coarsely chopped
6	carrots, sliced
2	cups water or vegetable stock
1	teaspoon curry powder
2	cups soymilk
½	teaspoon salt

Simmer chopped onion and carrots in a covered pot with the water and curry powder until the carrots can be easily pierced with a fork, about 20 minutes.

Puree the carrots and onions with their cooking water in a blender in two or three small batches, adding some of the soymilk to each batch to facilitate blending. Be sure to start the blender on low speed and hold the lid on tightly. The soup should be very smooth. If it seems too thick, add enough soymilk to achieve desired consistency. Return to the pot, add salt to taste and heat until steamy hot.

Serves 4

Nutrition information per serving:
105 calories (8% from fat); 3 g protein; 21 g carbohydrate; 1 g fat; 217 mg sodium; 87 mg calcium

Garden Vegetable Soup

1	onion, chopped
2	cloves garlic, minced
2	carrots, diced
1	stalk celery, sliced, including top
2	red potatoes, scrubbed and diced
1	15-ounce can crushed tomatoes
4	cups water
1½	teaspoons basil
1	teaspoon mixed Italian herbs
¼	teaspoon cumin
¼	teaspoon black pepper
2	medium zucchini, diced
1	15-ounce can kidney beans, including liquid
1	cup frozen corn
2	cups finely chopped kale

Prepare the onion, garlic, carrots, celery, and potatoes and place in a large pot with the crushed tomatoes and water. Stir in the Italian herbs, basil, and black pepper. Cover and simmer over medium heat until the carrots are just tender, about 15 minutes.

Add the zucchini, kidney beans with their liquid, corn, and chopped kale. Cover and simmer until the zucchini is just tender, about 10 minutes.

Serves 8

Nutrition information per serving:
127 calories (1.5% from fat); 3 g protein; 28 g carbohydrate; 0.2 g fat; 166 mg sodium; 65 mg calcium

Curried Lentil Soup

This simple soup is made in a single pot. Serve it with cooked greens and fresh bread.

1	cup lentils, rinsed
1	onion, chopped
2	celery stalks, sliced
4	cloves garlic, minced
1	teaspoon whole cumin seed
8	cups water
½	cup couscous or white basmati rice
1	cup chopped tomatoes
1½	teaspoons curry powder
1/8	teaspoon black pepper
1	teaspoon salt

Place lentils, onion, celery, garlic, cumin seed and water in a large pot. Bring to a simmer, then cover loosely and cook until the lentils are tender, about 50 minutes.

Stir in couscous or rice, chopped tomatoes, curry powder, and pepper. Continue cooking until couscous or rice is tender, about 10 minutes for coucous or 15 minutes for rice. Add salt to taste.

Serves 8

Nutrition information per serving:
111 calories (2% from fat); 6 g protein; 21 g carbohydrate; 0.2 g fat; 327 mg of sodium; 26 mg calcium

Creamy Lima Soup

This soup is quick and delicious. Use fresh basil and parsley if possible. They really make the soup.

1	onion, chopped
1	large garlic clove, minced
2½	cups water or vegetable stock
1	cup crushed tomatoes
2	cups shredded cabbage
1	tablespoon fresh basil (or 1 teaspoon dried basil)
1	15-ounce can lima beans, drained
¹/₈	teaspoon black pepper
1	cup soymilk
2	tablespoons chopped fresh parsley
½	teaspoon salt

Heat ½ cup of water in a large pot then add the onion and garlic and cook until the onion is soft, about 5 minutes. Add the tomatoes, cabbage, basil, lima beans, pepper and remaining water or stock. Simmer for 15 minutes.

Ladle about 3 cups of the soup into a blender, add soymilk and fresh parsley, and blend until smooth, using a low speed and holding the lid on tightly. Return it to the pot and heat gently (do not boil) until very hot and steamy.

Serves 4 to 6

Nutrition information per serving:
145 calories (5% from fat); 6 g protein; 28 g carbohydrate; 0.8 g fat; 308 mg sodium; 97 mg calcium

Quick Vegetable Ramen

Ramen soups contain quick-cooking dried noodles and a packet of flavorful seasoning broth. By adding your own fresh vegetables, you can quickly make a tasty, nutritious meal. Ramen soups come in a variety of flavors from natural food stores and many supermarkets. Select brands without animal products or added oil.

1	package ramen soup
1	cup chopped broccoli
1	green onion, sliced

Follow package instructions for cooking ramen: Bring water to a boil and add the broccoli along with the noodles. Cook until the noodles are tender, then stir in the seasoning packet and sliced green onion. Serve at once.

Serves 2

Nutrition information per serving:
85 calories (8% from fat); 3 g protein; 17 g carbohydrate; 0.8 g fat; 81 mg sodium; 13 mg calcium

Autumn Stew

Based on traditional Native American foods--squash, corn, and beans--this stew is perfect for an autumn feast. Serve it with warm bread and a crisp green salad.

½	cup water or vegetable stock
1	tablespoon lite soy sauce
1	onion, chopped
1	red bell pepper, diced
4	large cloves of garlic, minced
1	pound (about 4 cups) butternut squash
1	15-ounce can chopped tomatoes
1	cup water
2	teaspoons oregano
1	teaspoon chili powder
½	teaspoon cumin
¼	teaspoon black pepper
1	15-ounce can kidney beans
1½	cups corn, fresh or frozen

Heat water and soy sauce in a large pot, then add the onion, bell pepper, and garlic. Cook over medium heat until the onion is translucent and most of the water has evaporated.

Cut the squash in half and remove the seeds, then peel and cut it into ½-inch cubes. Add to the onion mixture along with the chopped tomatoes, water, oregano, chili powder, cumin, and pepper. Cover and simmer until the squash is just tender when pierced with a fork, about 20 minutes, then add the kidney beans with their liquid and the corn. Cook 5 minutes longer.

Serves 8

Nutrition information per serving:
132 calories (4% from fat); 5 g protein; 27 g carbohydrate; 0.5 g fat; 267 mg sodium; 44 mg calcium

Potato and Cabbage Soup

4	potatoes, peeled and diced
1	large onion, chopped
4	cups shredded cabbage
4	cups vegetable stock or water
1	cup soymilk or rice milk
½-1	teaspoon salt

Place the potatoes, onion, and cabbage in a large pot with the water or vegetable stock. Bring to a simmer and cook 15 minutes. Remove about 3 cups of the soup to a blender and add the soymilk or rice milk. Blend until smooth then return it to the pot and stir to mix. Add salt to taste.

Serves 6 to 8

Nutrition information per serving:
139 calories (2% from fat); 3 g protein; 31 g carbohydrate; 0.3 g fat; 292 mg sodium; 47 mg calcium

Black Bean Soup

This Latin American favorite is hearty, healthy, and very low in fat.

1	onion, chopped
3	garlic cloves, crushed
2	stalks celery, sliced
1	carrot, diced
1	potato, diced
2	cups vegetable stock or water
2	15-ounce cans black beans, undrained
1	teaspoon oregano
1	teaspoon cumin
1	tablespoon lemon juice

Place all ingredients except lemon juice into a large pot and bring to a simmer. Cover and cook 15 minutes. Remove about 3 cups of the soup to a blender and blend until smooth, using a low speed and holding the lid on tightly. Return it to the pot and stir in the lemon juice.

Serves 6

Nutrition information per serving:
138 calories (2% from fat); 6 g protein; 28 g carbohydrate; 0.3 g fat; 198 mg sodium; 43 mg calcium

SALADS AND DRESSINGS

Salad dressing recipes can be easily made fat-free by replacing the oil with water, vegetable stock, bean cooking liquid, or seasoned rice vinegar. This section contains recipes for fat-free dressings, as well as several fat-free salads.

Fat-free Dressing

Seasoned rice vinegar makes a simple, delicious dressing for salads and cooked vegetables. Any extra dressing will keep in the refrigerator for 2 to 3 weeks.

½   cup seasoned rice vinegar
1-2   teaspoons stone-ground or Dijon mustard
1   clove garlic, pressed

Whisk all ingredients together. Use as a dressing for salads and for steamed vegetables. Makes ½ cup

Nutrition information per 1 tablespoon:
14 calories (0% from fat); 0 9 protein; 3 g carbohydrate; 0 g fat; 310 mg sodium; 1 mg calcium

Simple Piquant Dressing

This dressing is slightly spicy with a south-of-the-border flair.

¼   cup seasoned rice vinegar
2   tablespoons tomato ketchup
1   teaspoon stone-ground mustard
1   clove garlic, minced
½   teaspoon paprika
¼   teaspoon oregano
¹/₈   teaspoon ground cumin

Whisk all ingredients together

Nutrition information per 1 tablespoon:
12 calories (0% from fat); 0 g protein; 3 g carbohydrate; 0 g fat; 210 mg sodium; 1.5 mg calcium

Balsamic Vinaigrette

Balsamic vinegar is a delicious wine vinegar from Italy with a mellow flavor that is perfect for salads.

2	tablespoons balsamic vinegar
2	tablespoons seasoned rice vinegar
2	tablespoons water
1-2	cloves garlic, crushed

Whisk all ingredients together.

Makes 1/3 cup

Nutrition information per 1 tablespoon:
6 calories (0% from fat); O g protein;1.5 g carbohydrate; O g fat; 99 mg sodium; 1 mg calcium

Curry Dressing

3	tablespoons seasoned rice vinegar
3	tablespoons water
2	teaspoons stone-ground or Dijon mustard
1	teaspoon lite soy sauce
1	teaspoon sugar or other sweetener
½	teaspoon curry powder
¼	teaspoon black pepper

Whisk all ingredients together.

Makes ½ cup

Nutrition information per 1 tablespoon:
9 calories (0% from fat); O g protein; 2 g carbohydrate; O g fat; 151 mg sodium; 1 mg calcium

Mixed Greens Salad

Prewashed mixtures of salad greens are available in most supermarkets and natural food stores. These mixes are as flavorful as they are attractive and make a satisfying salad with just a touch of dressing. Other vegetables can be added for additional flavor and nutrition, as the following recipe suggests.

½	red or yellow bell pepper, seeded and sliced
1	red or yellow tomato, sliced
½	cup peeled and sliced cucumber or jicama
6	cups prewashed salad mix
3	tablespoons fat-free dressing

Combine all ingredients and toss gently to mix. Top with your favorite fat-free dressing.

Serves 6

Nutrition information per serving:
20 calories (3% from fat); 0.2 g protein; 4 g carbohydrate; 0.1 9 fat; 160 mg sodium; 42 mg calcium

Four Bean Salad

This colorful salad is quick to prepare and keeps well.

1	15-ounce can dark kidney beans, drained
1	15-ounce can black-eye peas, drained
1	10-ounce package frozen lima beans, thawed
1	15-ounce can vegetarian chili beans or pinquitos, undrained
1	large red bell pepper, diced
½	cup finely chopped onion
2	cups corn, fresh or frozen
¼	cup seasoned rice vinegar
2	tablespoons apple cider or distilled vinegar
1	lemon, juiced

2   teaspoons cumin
1   teaspoon coriander
$^1/_8$ teaspoon cayenne

Drain the kidney beans, black-eye peas, and lima beans and combine in a large bowl. Add the pinquitos or chili beans, along with their sauce. Stir in the bell pepper, onion, and corn.

Whisk the remaining ingredients together and pour over the salad. Toss gently to mix. Chill at least 1 hour before serving, if possible.

Serves 10

Nutrition information per serving:
216 calories (2% from fat); 11 g protein; 41 g carbohydrate; 0.5 g fat; 104 mg sodium; 52 mg calcium

Quick and Colorful Couscous Salad

Couscous is actually a type of pasta which cooks almost instantly and makes a quick and beautiful salad.

1   cup couscous
1   cup boiling water
1   red bell pepper, diced
1   cucumber, peeled, seeded and diced
1   carrot, grated
¼   cup raisins or currants
2   tablespoons lemon juice
1   tablespoon cider vinegar
1   tablespoon apple juice concentrate
1   teaspoon stone-ground or Dijon mustard
½   teaspoon salt
½   teaspoon curry powder
¼   teaspoon cumin

Place couscous in a large bowl and pour boiling water over it. Stir just to mix, then cover and let stand 5 to 10 minutes. Fluff with a fork. Cool.

When the couscous is cool, add the diced bell pepper and cucumber, the grated carrot, and the raisins.

Mix the lemon juice, vinegar, apple juice concentrate, mustard and seasonings together and pour over salad. Toss to mix.

Serves 6

Nutrition information per serving:
117 calories (1% from fat); 3 g protein; 26 g carbohydrate; 0.2 g fat; 198 mg sodium; 16 mg calcium

Red Potato Salad

Red potatoes make a beautiful and delicious fat-free potato salad.

4	large red potatoes, scrubbed
1	small red onion, thinly sliced
1	red or yellow bell pepper, seeded and sliced
¼	cup finely chopped fresh parsley
¼	cup cider vinegar
¼	cup fresh lemon juice
2	tablespoons seasoned rice vinegar
2	cloves garlic, crushed
2	teaspoons stone-ground or Dijon mustard
¼-½	teaspoon black pepper

Cut the potatoes into ½-inch cubes and steam over boiling water until just tender, 10 to 15 minutes. Rinse with cold water, then place in a large bowl to cool. When the potatoes are cool, add the onion, bell pepper, and parsley. Combine the remaining ingredients for the dressing. Pour over salad and toss gently to mix. Serves 8

Variation: Substitute Yukon Gold potatoes, available in many markets, for the red potatoes.

Nutrition information per serving:
90 calories (2% from fat); 2 g protein; 20 g carbohydrate; 0.2 g fat; 124 mg of sodium; 17 mg calcium

Spinach Salad with Curry Dressing

This wonderful spinach salad is a happy marriage of flavors and textures. It is especially easy to make when you use prewashed fresh spinach available in the produce department of most markets.

1	bunch fresh spinach, washed or ½ bag prewashed spinach
1	green apple, diced
2	green onions, including green tops, finely sliced
¼	cup golden raisins
3	tablespoons seasoned rice vinegar
3	tablespoons frozen apple juice concentrate
2	teaspoons stone-ground or Dijon mustard
1	teaspoon lite soy sauce
½	teaspoon curry powder
¼	teaspoon black pepper

Combine the washed spinach with the apple, onions, and raisins in a large salad bowl. Whisk together the vinegar, apple juice concentrate, mustard, soy sauce, curry powder and black pepper in a small bowl. Pour over salad and toss to mix just before serving.

Serves 6 to 8

Nutrition information per serving:
45 calories (2% from fat); 1.3 g protein; 9 g carbohydrate; 0.1 g fat; 210 mg sodium; 65 mg calcium

Aztec Salad

This salad is a fiesta of color and taste. It may be made in advance, and keeps well for several days. If you are a cilantro lover, you may want to add a little extra.

2	15-ounce cans black beans
½	cup finely chopped red onion
1	green bell pepper, diced
1	red or yellow bell pepper, diced
2	tomatoes, diced
2	cups frozen corn, thawed
¾	cup chopped fresh cilantro (optional)
2	tablespoons seasoned rice vinegar
2	tablespoons apple cider or distilled vinegar
1	lime or lemon, juiced
2	garlic cloves, minced
2	teaspoons cumin
1	coriander
½	teaspoon crushed red pepper flakes, or a pinch of cayenne

Drain and rinse the beans and place them in a large salad bowl with the onion, peppers, tomatoes, corn, and cilantro. In a small bowl, combine the vinegars, garlic, lemon or lime juice and seasonings and pour over salad. Toss gently to mix.

Serves 10

Nutrition information per serving:
143 calories (2% from fat); 7 g protein; 30 g carbohydrate; 0.3 g fat; 171 mg sodium, 31 mg calcium

Pasta Salad

Using a commercial fat-free dressing makes this salad a snap to make. If you want to make your own dressing, use the Fat-free Dressing on page 128.

8	ounces uncooked pasta (spirals, shells, etc.)
1	cup fat-free Italian dressing (homemade or store bought)
1	cup cooked kidney beans, drained
1	cup cooked garbanzo beans, drained
1	red bell pepper, seeded and diced
3-4	green onions, sliced
1	15-ounce can water-packed artichoke hearts, drained (optional)

Cook the pasta in a large pot according to package directions until it is just tender. Rinse with cold water, then drain and place it into a large bowl. Pour the dressing over the pasta and stir to mix. Add all of the remaining ingredients and toss gently to mix.

Serves 8

Nutrition information per serving:
198 calories (3% from fat); 7 g protein; 40 g carbohydrate; 0.8 g fat; 157 mg sodium; 42 mg calcium

White Bean Salad

You'll love the tangy flavor of this super-easy salad.
1 15-ounce can white beans, drained and rinsed
1 small red bell pepper, diced

½	cup finely chopped parsley
2	tablespoons lemon juice (1 lemon)
2	teaspoons balsamic vinegar
¼	teaspoon garlic granules or garlic powder
¼	teaspoon black pepper

Combine all ingredients in a large bowl. Let stand 10 to 15 minutes before serving if possible.

Serves 4 to 6

Nutrition information per serving:
103 calories (2% from fat); 6 g protein; 19 g carbohydrate; 0.2 g fat; 184 mg sodium; 63 mg calcium

Cucumber Salad

This salad is colorful, quick to make, and keeps well. It is particularly cool and appealing with chili, curries, and other spicy foods.

3	cucumbers
2	tomatoes
½	small red onion
½	teaspoon basil
½	teaspoon dill weed
1	tablespoon chopped fresh parsley
	apple cider vinegar

Peel the cucumbers, slice them in half lengthwise, and scoop out the seeds. Cut the cucumber into bite-sized pieces. Dice the tomatoes, and finely chop the red onion. Toss the vegetables together, then sprinkle with basil, dill, and fresh parsley. Add enough vinegar to coat all the vegetables, and toss to mix. Chill before serving if possible

Serves 6

Nutrition information per serving:
35 calories (4% from fat); 1 g protein; 7 g carbohydrate; 0.2 g fat; 7 mg sodium, 28 mg calcium

VEGETABLES

Broccoli with Fat-free Dressing

You'll love broccoli when it's served with this delicious fat-free dressing that is easy to make, keeps well in the refrigerator, and is tasty on other vegetables as well.

1	bunch broccoli
¼	cup seasoned rice vinegar
1	teaspoon stone-ground or Dijon mustard
1	clove garlic, pressed or minced

Break the broccoli into bite-sized florets. Peel the stems and slice them into ¼-inch thick rounds. Steam until just tender, about 3 minutes.

While the broccoli is steaming, whisk the dressing ingredients in a serving bowl. Add the steamed broccoli and toss to mix. Serve immediately. 4 to 6 servings

Nutrition information per serving:
32 calories (4% from fat); 1.5 g protein; 6 g carbohydrate; 0.2 g fat; 216 mg sodium; 88 mg calcium

Braised Cabbage

This simple cooking technique brings out the delicious, sweet flavor of cabbage.

½	cup water
2	cups cabbage, coarsely chopped
	salt and fresh ground black pepper

Bring water to a boil in a skillet or saucepan. Stir in cabbage, cover and cook until it is just tender, about 5 minutes. Sprinkle with salt and pepper to taste. Serves 2 to 3

Nutrition information per serving:
16 calories (0% from fat); 0.5 g protein; 4 g carbohydrate;0 g fat; 80 mg of sodium; 33 mg calcium

Simply Wonderful Winter Squash

In spite of its name, winter squash is available year round in most places. If you've never tried a butternut, or kabocha, or delicata you're in for a real treat. Try this easy recipe for starters.

1	winter squash (butternut, kabocha, delicata, etc.)
½-1	cup water
1-2	teaspoons lite soy sauce
1	tablespoon maple syrup

Peel the winter squash and remove the seeds. Cut the squash into 1-inch cubes (you should have about 4 cups) and place it into a large pot with the water, soy sauce, and maple syrup. Cover and simmer over medium heat until the squash is fork tender.

Makes 4 cups

Nutrition information per 1 cup:
92 calories (6% from fat); 2 g protein; 19 g carbohydrate; 1 g fat; 102 mg sodium; 33 mg calcium

Steamed Kale

Kale is an excellent source of calcium and beta-carotene, and simply delicious when prepared according to the recipe below. The secret to really delicious kale is to choose young, tender greens.

1   bunch (about 1 pound) kale
½   cup water
1   teaspoon lite soy sauce
2-3   cloves garlic, minced

Wash the kale, remove the stems and chop the leaves into half-inch wide strips. Heat the water and soy sauce in a large pot or skillet and add the garlic. Cook 30 seconds, then add the greens, toss to mix, cover and cook over medium-low heat for 3 to 5 minutes. Add water, 1 tablespoon at a time, if necessary to keep the greens from sticking.

Makes 2 cups

Nutrition information per ½ cup:
61 calories (6% from fat); 3 g protein; 11 g carbohydrate; 0.4 g fat; 101 mg sodium; 158 mg calcium

Green Beans with Sweet Onions

Green beans take on a slightly Asian flair in this simple recipe.

1   pound fresh green beans (about 3 cups)
¼   cup water
1   tablespoon lite soy sauce
1   tablespoon seasoned rice vinegar
1   medium-small yellow onion, thinly sliced

Trim beans and break into bite-sized pieces. Steam until just tender, about 10 minutes.

In a large skillet, heat water, soy sauce, and seasoned rice vinegar. Add the sliced onion and cook over medium heat until onion is soft, 3 to 5 minutes. Lower heat and continue cooking until most of the liquid is evaporated and onion is lightly browned and sweet. Add steamed beans, toss and serve.

Serves 6

Nutrition information per serving:
36 calories (0% from fat); 2 g protein; 7 g carbohydrate; 0 g fat; 105 mg sodium; 36 mg calcium

Roasted Yams or Sweet Potatoes

4   yams or sweet potatoes
1   teaspoon each: garlic powder and mixed Italian herbs
¼   teaspoon salt
     fresh ground black pepper

Preheat oven to 500°. Scrub the sweet potatoes or yams and cut them into chunks. Spray a 9 x 13-inch baking dish with nonstick spray. Spread the yams in the dish, sprinkle with the seasonings, and toss to mix. Bake until tender when pierced with a fork, 25 to 30 minutes.

Serves 6

Nutrition information per serving:
158 calories (0% from fat); 1.5 g protein; 38 g carbohydrate; 0 g fat; 100 mg sodium; 19 mg calcium

Oven Fries

Great fries without the grease!

4 medium large potatoes
2 teaspoon each: garlic powder and mixed Italian herbs
½ teaspoon paprika
fresh ground black pepper

Preheat oven to 500°. Scrub the potatoes and cut them into strips. Lightly spray a 9 x 1 3-inch baking dish with nonstick spray and spread the potatoes in it. Sprinkle with the seasonings, and toss to mix. Bake until tender when pierced with a fork, about 30 minutes.

Serves 6

Nutrition information per serving:
147 calories (0.5% from fat); 2 g protein; 34 g carbohydrate; 0.1 g fat; 100 mg sodium; 14 mg calcium

Golden Potatoes

Top these colorful, spicy potatoes with chutney, and serve them with lentil or bean soups.

4	large red potatoes
2	teaspoons whole mustard seed
½	teaspoon turmeric
½	teaspoon cumin
¼	teaspoon ginger
$1/_8$	teaspoon cayenne
$1/_8$	teaspoon black pepper
1	cup water onion, chopped
1 ½	teaspoons lite soy sauce

Scrub the potatoes, then cut them into ½-inch cubes and steam them until tender when pierced with a fork, 20 to 25 minutes. Cool thoroughly.

Toast the spices in a large nonstick skillet for 1 to 2 minutes, then carefully pour in ½ cup of the water. Add the chopped onion and cook, stirring frequently, until the onion is soft and most of the liquid has evaporated, about 5 minutes. Add the cooled potatoes along with the remaining water and the soy sauce. Stir to mix, then cover and cook over medium heat for 5 minutes. Stir before serving.

Serves 6

Nutrition information per serving:
161 calories (1% from fat); 3 g protein; 37 g carbohydrate; 0.1 g fat; 62 mg of sodium; 24 mg calcium

GRAINS

Brown Rice

Cooking brown rice in extra water ensures perfect rice every time, and actually reduces the cooking time. Roasting makes this brown rice delicious.

1 cup short grain brown rice
3 cups water
½ teaspoon salt, optional

Rinse the rice in a saucepan, then drain. Put the pan of drained, but still wet, rice on a burner, set it to medium-high heat, and stir constantly until the rice dries, about one minute. This toasts the rice. Stop when the rice is thoroughly dried--we are not making popcorn. Then add water, bring to a boil, cover, and simmer 35-40 minutes, until the rice is soft but still retains a hint of crunchiness. Do not overcook. Pour off the remaining water. Serve with beans, vegetables, curry, or a dash of low-sodium soy sauce.

Makes 3 cups of cooked rice

Nutrition information per ½ cup:
115 calories (4% from fat); 2.5 g protein; 25 g carbohydrate; 0.5 g fat; 176 mg sodium; 13 mg calcium

Quick Confetti Rice

This colorful rice pilaf has no added fat, so be sure to use a nonstick skillet.

2 cups cooked brown rice
2 tablespoons water or stock
½ cup frozen corn
½ cup frozen peas
½ cup diced red bell pepper, fresh or canned
½ teaspoon curry powder
¼ cup raisins (optional)
  salt to taste

Add water to skillet, along with cooked rice. Using a spatula or the back of a wooden spoon, separate the rice kernels. Add remaining ingredients and heat until steamy hot. Add salt to taste.

Makes about 3 cups

Nutrition information per ½ cup:
109 calories (3% from fat); 2.5 g protein; 24 g carbohydrate; 0.3 g fat; 112 mg sodium; 14 mg calcium

Bulgur

Bulgur is cracked wheat which has been toasted to give it a delicious, nutty flavor. It cooks in about 15 minutes and is an excellent accompaniment to a wide variety of foods, from chili to roasted vegetables.

2	cups water
1	cup bulgur
½	teaspoon salt

Bring water to a boil in a saucepan, then stir in bulgur and salt. Reduce heat to a simmer, then cover and cook until bulgur is tender, about 15 minutes.

Makes about 2 ½ cups

Nutrition information per ½ cup:
113 calories (2% from fat); 4 g protein; 24 g carbohydrate; 0.2 g fat; 216 mg sodium; 14 mg calcium

Spanish Bulgur

Cracked and toasted wheat makes a quick and delicious Spanish pilaf. Serve it with chili or refried beans.

1	cup bulgur wheat
1 ¾	cups boiling water
2	teaspoons lite soy sauce
1	teaspoon garlic granules
$^2/_3$	teaspoons chili powder
½	teaspoon ground cumin
¼	teaspoon salt

Place the bulgur in a large bowl and pour the boiling water over it. Cover the bowl and let stand 30 minutes, until bulgur is tender. Pour the bulgur into a large skillet and add the remaining ingredients. Turn with a spatula to mix in the spices, and continue cooking until the mixture is very hot. Serve immediately. Makes 2 ½ cups

Nutrition information per ½ cup:
100 calories (2% from fat); 4 g protein; 21 g carbohydrate; 0.2 g fat; 167 mg of sodium; 14 mg calcium

Couscous

Couscous cooks in minutes and makes a delicious side dish or salad.

1½	cups boiling water
½	teaspoon salt
1	cup couscous

Bring salted water to a boil in a small pan. Stir in the couscous, then remove the pan from heat and cover it. Let stand 10 to 15 minutes, then fluff with a fork and serve. Makes 3 cups

Nutrition information per ½ cup:
91 calories (0% from fat); 3 g protein; 20 g carbohydrate; 0 g fat; 93 mg sodium; 1 mg calcium

Polenta

Polenta, or coarsely ground cornmeal, has long been a staple grain in northern Italy. It cooks easily and is delicious with marinara or any other spicy sauce. Pour the cooked polenta onto a platter and top it with sauce, or spoon it into a bread pan and chill, then slice and grill it.

1	cup polenta
1	cup cold water
½-1	teaspoon salt
4	cups boiling water

Stir polenta and cold water together in a saucepan. Stir in salt and boiling water and simmer, stirring frequently, until thickened, about 15 minutes.

Makes 4 cups

Nutrition information per 1/2 cup:
62 calories (3% from fat); 1.5 g protein; 14 g carbohydrate; 0.2 g fat; 267 mg sodium; 2 mg calcium

MAIN DISHES

Pasta with Roasted Summer Vegetables

What a happy coincidence that the easiest way to cook vegetables is also the tastiest. Oven-roasting vegetables takes only minutes and brings out their very best flavor.

3	summer squash (zucchini, crookneck, etc.)
1	large red onion
1	large red bell pepper, seeded
2	cups small, firm mushrooms
½	pound very firm tofu, cut into 1-inch cubes (optional)
1	teaspoon garlic granules
1	teaspoon mixed Italian herbs
1	teaspoon chili powder
½	teaspoon salt
¼	teaspoon black pepper
12	ounces pasta, preferably whole grain
2	tomatoes, cut into wedges

Preheat the oven to 500°. Cut the squash, red onion, and bell pepper into generous 1-inch chunks and place in a large bowl. Clean the mushrooms and add them to the bowl. Gently mix in the tofu cubes if desired. Sprinkle with the garlic granules, Italian herbs, chili powder, salt, and pepper and toss gently to mix. Spread the vegetables in a single layer in one or two baking dishes and bake in the preheated oven until tender, about 10 minutes.

Cook the pasta according to package instructions. Rinse quickly with cold water and place on a large plate or platter. Top with the roasted vegetables and the fresh tomato wedges. Serve immediately. Serves 6 to 8

Nutrition information per serving:
172 calories (8% from fat); 10 g protein; 29 g carbohydrate; 1.5 g fat; 84 mg sodium; 72 mg calcium.

Very Primo Pasta

Mix up some pasta with vegetables and beans for a delicious meal.

½	cup water or vegetable stock
1	onion, chopped
1	bell pepper, diced
1	carrot, sliced
1	stalk of celery, sliced
2	cups sliced mushrooms
1	15-ounce can crushed or chopped tomatoes
1	15-ounce can kidney beans, drained
1	teaspoon basil
½	teaspoon paprika
½	teaspoon black pepper
1	tablespoon lite soy sauce
8	ounces pasta spirals or shells

In a large pot, heat the water or stock. Cook the onions for 3 minutes, then add the pepper, carrots, and celery and cook for 5 minutes over medium heat. Add the mushrooms, then cover the pan and cook an additional 7 minutes, stirring occasionally. Add the tomatoes, kidney beans, basil, paprika, pepper, and soy sauce, then cover and cook 10 to 15 minutes.

Cook pasta in a large pot of boiling water until just tender. Rinse and drain, then stir it into the vegetable mixture to serve.

Serves 8

Nutrition information per serving:
147 calories (2% from fat); 6.5 g protein; 29 g carbohydrate; 0.4 g fat; 77 mg of sodium; 38 mg calcium

Super Chili

A big batch of this delicious chili made on Sunday is great for quick reheating later in the week. Always a hit. This recipe uses textured vegetable protein (TVP), which has the taste and texture of ground beef with none of the fat. It is available at all health food stores.

1	28-ounce can crushed tomatoes
1	3-ounce can tomato paste
1	large onion, chopped
1	green pepper, chopped
1	cup textured vegetable protein
1	cup water
1	jalapeno pepper, minced
2	tablespoons (or more) chili powder
1	teaspoon cumin
2	teaspoons garlic powder
1	teaspoon oregano
¼	teaspoon allspice
1	15-ounce can red kidney beans

Combine all ingredients, except for kidney beans, in a large saucepan or Dutch oven. Cover pan and simmer for 30 minutes. Taste and add salt if needed. Then add kidney beans. Return to a boil, and serve. Serve on hot rice or, for an interesting switch, on top of spaghetti.

Serves 6

Nutrition analysis per serving:
155 calories (3% from fat); 12 g protein; 25 g carbohydrate; 0.5g fat; 370 mg sodium; 88 mg calcium

Quick Chili

There's nothing quite like a bowl of steaming hot chili to warm a cold winter day. Textured vegetable protein (TVP), which adds flavor and texture, is available in natural food stores.

1	cup water or vegetable stock
1	onion, chopped
1	green bell pepper, diced
2	large garlic cloves, minced
½	cup textured vegetable protein
1	15-ounce cans pinto beans
1	15-ounce can tomato sauce
1	cup corn, fresh or frozen
1-2	teaspoons chili powder
1	teaspoon oregano
½	teaspoon ground cumin
$1/_8$	teaspoon cayenne (more for spicier beans)

Heat 1 cup of water or stock in a large pot and cook the onion, bell pepper, and garlic until the onion is soft, about 5 minutes. Add the remaining ingredients and simmer at least 30 minutes.

Serves 8

Nutrition information per serving:
164 calories (2% from fat); 10 g protein; 30 g carbohydrate; 0.4 g fat; 158 mg sodium; 73 mg calcium

Quick Chili Corn Pie

This is a delicious casserole with spicy beans on the bottom, and cornbread on the top.

1½	cups soymilk
1½	tablespoons vinegar
2	15-ounce cans vegetarian chili beans, with their juice
1	10-ounce package frozen corn
1	cup corn meal
1	teaspoon baking soda
¼	teaspoon salt

Mix the soymilk and vinegar and set aside. Spread the chili beans in a 9 x 9-inch casserole then stir in the corn. Place bean mixture in the oven and turn it on to 400°.

In a bowl, combine the corn meal, baking soda, and salt. Stir in the soymilk mixture. When the oven reaches 400°, remove the bean mixture (remember to use potholders!). Pour the cornmeal batter over the beans and return it to the oven to bake until the bread is set and golden brown, about 30 minutes.

Serves 8

Nutrition information per serving:
234 calories (14% from fat); 9 g protein; 41 g carbohydrate; 4 g fat; 329 mg sodium; 28 mg calcium

Fiesta Plate

In this dish, pinto beans are cooked with garlic and cumin, and served on brown rice with a green salad on top for a delicious and satisfying meal.
Beans:

3	15-ounce cans pinto beans
4	large garlic cloves, minced
1½	teaspoons whole cumin seed

1	cup water
½	teaspoon salt

Place the beans with their liquid in a large pot with the garlic, cumin, and water. Simmer for 20 minutes.

Rice:

3	cups water
½	teaspoon salt (optional)
1	cup brown rice

Bring water to a boil, and add salt if desired, then sprinkle in the rice. Cover and simmer over medium heat until the rice is just tender, about 40 minutes. Pour off any excess water.

Salad:

1	bunch leaf lettuce
1	cucumber, sliced
1	tomato, diced
½	cup diced jicama (optional)

Dressing:

¼	cup seasoned rice vinegar
1	teaspoon stone-ground or Dijon mustard
1	clove garlic, pressed

Wash and dry the lettuce, and tear it into bite sized pieces. Add the cucumber, tomato, and cabbage. Whisk the vinegar, mustard and garlic together for the dressing and toss with the salad.

To serve, place a generous spoonful of rice on each plate and top with beans and some of their liquid. Serve the salad on top of the beans or to the side.

Serves 8

Nutrition information per serving:
176 calories (3% from fat); 6 g protein; 35 g carbohydrate;1 g fat; 293 mg sodium; 63 mg calcium

Spicy Indonesian Stir Fry

Once the vegetables are all prepared, this dish cooks in a flash. Udon is a Japanese pasta available in many supermarkets and natural food stores. If you cannot find it, use spaghetti.

8	ounces spaghetti or udon noodles
½	cup water or vegetable stock
1	onion, sliced
2	cups sliced mushrooms
½	pound firm tofu, cut into cubes
2	stalks celery, sliced
2	cups shredded green cabbage
1	red bell pepper, seeded and cut into strips
2	cups bean sprouts (optional)
1	teaspoon turmeric
½	teaspoon cumin
¼	teaspoon cayenne
2	tablespoons lite soy sauce

Cut up the vegetables as indicated above. Then cook the noodles in a large pot of boiling water until just tender. Drain and rinse quickly with cold water.

Heat the water or stock in a large nonstick wok or skillet, then add the onion and cook over medium-high heat until soft, about 3 minutes. Add the mushrooms, tofu, and celery and cook another 3 minutes. Add the cabbage and bell pepper, then cover and cook 4 minutes, stirring occasionally. Stir in the spices and soy sauce, then add the cooked noodles and toss gently to mix. Serve immediately.

Serves 8

Nutrition information per serving:
107 calories (8% from fat); 7 g protein; 17 g carbohydrate; 1 g fat; 172 mg of sodium; 70 mg calcium

Shepherd's Pie

This is a hearty and satisfying vegetable stew with a top "crust" of fluffy mashed potatoes.

4	large russet potatoes, diced
½-1	cup soymilk
½	teaspoon salt
½	cup water or vegetable stock
2	onions, chopped
1	large bell pepper, diced
2	carrots, sliced
2	stalks of celery, sliced
½	pound (about 2 cups) mushrooms, sliced
1	15-ounce can chopped tomatoes
1	15-ounce can kidney beans, drained
½	teaspoon paprika
½	teaspoon black pepper
2	tablespoons lite soy sauce

Dice the potatoes and steam them until tender. Mash, adding enough soymilk to make them smooth and spreadable. Add salt to taste. Set aside.

In a large pot, heat the water or stock and cook the onions for 3 minutes. Add the pepper, carrots, and celery and cook for 5 minutes over medium heat. Add the mushrooms, then cover the pan and cook an additional 7 minutes, stirring occasionally. Add the tomatoes, kidney beans, paprika, pepper and soy sauce, then cover and cook 10 to 15 minutes.

Put the vegetables into a 9 x 13-inch baking dish and spread the mashed potatoes evenly over the top. Sprinkle with paprika. Bake at 350° for 25 minutes, until hot and bubbly. Serves 8

Nutrition information per serving:
272 calories (2% from fat); 8 g protein; 58 g carbohydrate; 0.5 g fat; 301 mg sodium; 63 mg calcium

Spinach and Mushroom Fritatta

This fritatta is like a crustless quiche. It is made with silken tofu, which is available in most grocery stores and all health food stores.

½	cup water
1	onion, chopped
2	cloves garlic, minced
2	cups sliced mushrooms
1	10-ounce package frozen spinach, thawed and squeezed dry
1	10.5-ounce package firm silken tofu
2	teaspoons dried basil
½	teaspoon salt
¼	teaspoon black pepper
¼	teaspoon nutmeg
¼	teaspoon celery seed
2	tablespoons couscous
¼	cup soymilk, rice milk, or water
1	ripe tomato, thinly sliced

Preheat oven to 350°. Heat water in a large pot or skillet and cook onion and garlic until soft, about 3 minutes. Add mushrooms and cook another 5 minutes. Stir in spinach and cook until mixture is very dry.

In a food processor or blender, process tofu and tahini until very smooth. Rub the basil between the palms of your hands to crush it, then mix it into the tofu, along with the salt, pepper, nutmeg, celery seed, couscous and soymilk. Add to the spinach mixture and stir to mix.

Pour into a 10-inch pie pan which has been sprayed with a nonstick spray. Bake for 15 minutes. Arrange sliced tomatoes around the edge, then bake another 10 minutes. Let stand 10 minutes before serving. Serves 8

Nutrition information per serving:
72 calories (9% from fat); 5 g protein; 11 g carbohydrate; 1 g fat; 269 mg sodium; 91 mg calcium

Lasagne

This delicious lasagne was adapted from a recipe given to me by my friend Gail Davis. You'll love how easy it is to make.

2	10-ounce packages of frozen chopped spinach, thawed
1	pound soft tofu
1	pound firm tofu
1	tablespoon basil
2	teaspoons garlic powder
1	teaspoon salt
¼	cup soymilk or rice milk
2	tablespoons lemon juice
1	tablespoon maple syrup
1	32-ounce jar marinara or 4 cups homemade sauce
8	ounces lasagne noodles (about 10 noodles), uncooked
½	cup water

Squeeze the spinach as dry as possible and set aside.

Process the tofu, garlic powder, basil, salt, milk, lemon juice, and maple syrup in a food processor until smooth.

Preheat oven to 350°. Cover the bottom of a 9 x 13-inch baking dish with a thin layer of the marinara, then with a layer of the uncooked noodles. Top this with half of the tofu mixture, half of the spinach, and half of the remaining marinara. Repeat with noodles and the remaining tofu mixture and spinach. Top with the remaining sauce.

Cover tightly with foil and bake for 45 minutes. Let stand a few minutes before serving.

Serves 8

Nutrition Information per serving:
252 calories (11% from fat); 17 g protein; 38 g carbohydrate; 3 g fat; 506 mg sodium; 249 mg calcium

SANDWICHES, SPREADS, AND QUICK MEALS

Missing Egg Sandwich

This sandwich looks and tastes like egg salad, but without the cholesterol and saturated fat.

1	cup firm tofu (½ pound), mashed
1	green onion, finely chopped
2	tablespoons pickle relish
2	teaspoons stone-ground or Dijon mustard
¼	teaspoon each: cumin, turmeric, garlic powder
8	slices whole wheat bread
4	lettuce leaves
4	tomato slices

Combine all ingredients and mix thoroughly. Serve on whole wheat bread with lettuce and tomato.

Makes 4 sandwiches

Nutrition information per sandwich:
188 calories (17% from fat); 10 g protein; 28 g carbohydrate; 3.5 g fat; 246 mg sodium; 109 mg calcium

Quick Pita Sandwich

Pita bread makes a quick and easy sandwich. Look for it in your supermarket or natural food store.

1	15-ounce can garbanzo beans, drained
1	stalk celery, finely sliced
1	green onion, finely chopped
2	teaspoons stone-ground mustard
1	tablespoon sweet pickle relish
6	pita breads
6	lettuce leaves, shredded
2	small tomatoes, diced

Mash the garbanzo beans with a fork or potato masher. Leave some chunks. Add the sliced celery, chopped onion, mustard, and relish. Cut the tops off the pita bread and open up the pockets. Use a spoon to stuff each pocket with a generous amount of the garbanzo mixture, then garnish with lettuce and tomatoes.

Makes 6 sandwiches

Nutrition information per serving:
213 calories (10% from fat); 8.5 g protein; 38 g carbohydrate; 2 g fat; 323 mg sodium; 87 mg calcium

Quick Black Bean Burritos

Burritos are quick and tasty, and can be eaten hot or cold. This one is made with black beans, but you could also use refried pinto beans. Handy bean flakes and fat-free refried beans are available in natural food stores and many supermarkets.

1	cup black bean flakes mixed with 1 cup boiling water or
1	15-ounce can fat-free refried black beans, heated
4	flour tortillas
1-2	cups shredded lettuce
2-3	tomatoes, sliced
3	green onions, sliced
1	cup salsa

Heat a tortilla in a large, ungreased skillet until it is warm and soft. Spread a line of black beans down the center of the tortilla, then top with lettuce, tomato, onions, and salsa. Fold the bottom end toward the center, then roll the tortilla around the filling. Repeat with remaining tortillas.

Makes 4 burritos

Nutrition information per burrito:
300 calories (10% from fat); 12 g protein; 55 g carbohydrate; 3 g fat; 196 mg sodium; 82 mg calcium

Terrific Tacos

Textured vegetable protein (TVP) is made from soybeans and makes a quick and tasty taco filling. It is available in natural food stores and some supermarkets. The recipe makes enough filling for 12 tacos. If this is more than you need for a particular meal, refrigerate any extra filling and garnishes for almost-instant future meals.

1	cup water
1	small onion, chopped
1	small green bell pepper, diced
¾	cup dry textured vegetable protein
1	cup tomato sauce
2	teaspoons chili powder
1	teaspoon garlic granules or powder
½	teaspoon cumin
¼	teaspoon oregano
1	tablespoon lite soy sauce
12	corn tortillas
1	cup shredded leaf lettuce
1	medium tomato, diced
4	green onions, sliced
½	cup salsa or taco sauce

Heat the water in a large pan then add the onion and bell pepper and cook for 5 minutes. Add the TVP, tomato sauce, chili powder, garlic, cumin, oregano, nutritional yeast, and soy sauce. Cook over low heat until the TVP is softened and the mixture is fairly dry, about 8 minutes.

Heat a tortilla in a heavy, ungreased skillet, flipping it from side to side until it is soft and pliable. Place a small amount of filling in the center, fold the tortilla in half, and cook each side for 1 minute. Garnish with lettuce, onions, tomatoes, and salsa.

Makes 10 to 12 tacos

Nutrition information per taco:
126 calories (10 % from fat); 7 g protein; 21 g carbohydrate; 1 g fat; 75 mg of sodium; 92 mg calcium

Quick Bean Tacos

Bean tacos are quick and easy, whether you're making one or two for an individual meal or many for a ravenous crowd.

1	15-ounce can fat-free refried beans, heated
8	corn tortillas

Garnishes: salsa
shredded leaf lettuce
green onions
diced tomatoes

Spread the tortilla with a thin layer (about ¼ cup) of refried beans and lay it flat (with the beans facing up) in an ungreased skillet over medium heat. When the tortilla becomes warm and pliable, fold it in half and cook each side for 1 minute. Garnish with salsa, lettuce, onions and tomatoes. Refrigerate the extra refried beans in an airtight plastic container for future use.

Enough for 8 tacos

Nutrition information per taco:
124 calories (9% from fat); 5 g protein; 23 g carbohydrate; 1 g fat; 151 mg sodium; 186 mg calcium

Pita Pizzas

Pita pizzas are quick and easy to prepare for meals or for snacks. You can make them almost instantly if you keep some pizza sauce and chopped vegetables in the refrigerator.

1	jar pizza sauce OR make your own sauce by mixing together:
1	15 ounce can tomato sauce
1	6 ounce can tomato paste
1	teaspoon garlic powder
½	teaspoon each: basil, oregano, and thyme
1	package pita bread
2	cups chopped vegetables: green onion, bell pepper, mushrooms

Turn pita bread upside down so it looks like a saucer. Spread with pizza sauce, then top liberally with chopped vegetables. Place on a cookie sheet and bake at 375° until the edges are lightly browned, about 10 minutes.

Note: You will only need about half the sauce for 6 pizzas. Refrigerate or freeze the remainder for use at another time.

Makes 6 pizzas

Nutrition information per pizza:
185 calories (9% from fat); 7 g protein; 35 g carbohydrate; 2 g fat; 337 mg sodium; 76 mg calcium

Crostini with Sun-Dried Tomatoes

In this fat-free version of crostini, thin slices of toasted bread are topped with a flavorful blend of tomatoes and roasted red peppers. You'll find sun-dried tomatoes in the dried fruit section of many markets. Roasted red peppers packed in water are usually found near the pickles and olives.

6	sun dried tomato halves
$2/3$	cup roasted red peppers (about 2 peppers)
1	garlic clove, crushed
1	tablespoon fresh basil, finely chopped or 1 teaspoon dried basil
$1/8$	teaspoon black pepper
1	baguette or Italian loaf, cut into ½-inch thick slices

Pour boiling water over the tomatoes and set aside until softened, about 30 minutes. Pour off the water (it can be saved and used in place of vegetable stock in other recipes), and coarsely chop the tomatoes. Chop the roasted red peppers and add to the tomatoes, along with the garlic, basil, pepper and salt. Let stand 30 minutes.

Place the bread on a baking sheet and toast in a 350° oven until outside is crisp, 10 to 15 minutes. Remove from the oven and cool slightly, then spread each piece with the tomato mixture.

Makes 20 slices

Nutrition Information per slice:
93 calories (1% from fat); 3 g protein; 18.5 g carbohydrate; 0.1 g fat; 179 mg sodium; 11 mg calcium

Beanie Weenies

Several companies make ready-to-eat vegetarian baked beans. Bush's and Heinz are two of the most widely available. Heat them with sliced vegetarian hot dogs, available at any health food store and many regular groceries, for a very-low-fat version of this old campfire favorite.

1	15-ounce can vegetarian baked beans
2	vegetarian hot dogs (Smart Dogs, Yves Veggie Wieners, etc.)

Place the beans in a medium saucepan. Slice the hot dogs into ¼-inch thick rounds and add them to the beans. Heat until bubbly.

Serves 2 to 3.

Nutrition information per serving:
134 calories (2% from fat); 10 g protein; 22 g carbohydrate; 0.3 g fat; 569 mg sodium; 54 mg calcium

Cheesy Garbanzo Spread

This spread has look and taste of spreadable cheese and takes only seconds to prepare. Try it on bread, crackers, or pasta. Look for jars of water-packed roasted red peppers near the pickles and olives at the grocery store.

1	15-ounce can garbanzo beans
½	cup roasted red peppers
3	tablespoons tahini (sesame seed butter)
3	tablespoons lemon juice

Drain beans, reserving liquid, and place in a food processor with the remaining ingredients. Process until very smooth. If the mixture is too thick, add a bit of garbanzo liquid.

Makes 2 cups

Nutrition information per ¼-cup serving:
125 calories (25% from fat); 5 g protein; 18 g carbohydrate; 3.5 g fat; 75 mg sodium; 30 mg calcium.

DESSERTS

Berry Cobbler

This delicious cobbler is quick and easy and may be prepared with fresh or frozen berries. Try raspberries, blackberries, boysenberries, blueberries, or a combination of these.

²/₃	cup whole wheat pastry flour
½	cup sugar or other sweetener
1½	teaspoons baking powder
¼	teaspoon salt
²/₃	cup soymilk or rice milk
1	20-ounce package frozen berries (about 2 ½ cups)

Preheat oven to 350°. In a mixing bowl, stir together the flour, sugar, baking power, and salt, then add the milk and stir until the batter is smooth.

Spread berries evenly in a 9 x 9-inch baking dish, then pour the batter over them. Bake at 350° for 45 minutes, until lightly browned.

Serves 8

Nutrition information per serving:
107 calories (2.5% from fat); 2 g protein; 24 g carbohydrate; 0.3 g fat; 77 mg sodium; 76 mg calcium.

Cranberry Apple Crisp

This fat-free dessert is colorful and easy to prepare. Using dried cranberries, you can make it any time of year. You'll find them in any market with a good dried fruit selection.

2	large green apples, peeled and sliced
½	cup fresh or dried cranberries
¾	cup rolled oats
¾	cups Grape-Nuts cereal

½   teaspoon cinnamon
⅓   cup maple syrup
⅔   cup apple juice
¼   teaspoon cornstarch or arrowroot

Preheat oven to 350°. Spread apple slices in a 9 x 9-inch baking dish. Sprinkle with cranberries.

In a mixing bowl, stir the oats, Grape-Nuts, and cinnamon together, then add the maple syrup and mix thoroughly. Distribute evenly over apple-cranberry mixture.

Mix apple juice with cornstarch or arrowroot, stirring to remove any lumps. Pour evenly over other ingredients. Bake for 45 minutes, or until apples are tender.

Serves 8

Nutrition information per serving:
139 calories (4% from fat); 2.5 g protein; 31 g carbohydrate; 0.6 g fat; 74 mg sodium; 24 mg calcium

Tropical Delight

Pureed frozen fruit makes a wonderful dessert, without the fat or refined sugar of ice cream. Many supermarkets carry frozen pineapple and mango, or you can make your own by freezing canned pineapple chunks and fresh mango. To freeze bananas, peel and break into chunks. Freeze in a single layer on a tray, then store in an airtight container.

1   orange, peeled
½   cup frozen banana chunks
1   cup frozen pineapple chunks
1   cup frozen mango chunks
½-1   cup soymilk or rice milk

Cut orange in half and remove any seeds, then place in a

blender with the remaining ingredients and process until thick and very smooth.

Serves 3

Nutrition information per serving:
152 calories (5% from fat); 2 g protein; 33 g carbohydrate; 1 g fat; 24 mg sodium; 54 mg calcium

Quick Rice Pudding

1½	cups soymilk (vanilla or plain)
1	tablespoon cornstarch or arrowroot
2	cups cooked rice (white or brown)
¼	cup maple syrup
¹/₃	cup raisins
¼	teaspoon cinnamon
1	teaspoon vanilla
½	teaspoon almond extract

Pour soymilk into a medium-sized saucepan and stir in cornstarch. Add rice, maple syrup, raisins and cinnamon and bring to a simmer over medium heat. Cook 3 minutes, then remove from heat and stir in vanilla and almond extract. Serve hot or cold.

Serves 3 to 4

Nutrition information per serving:
151 calories (6% from fat); 2.5 g protein; 34 g carbohydrate; 1 g fat; 28 mg sodium; 46 mg calcium

Bread Pudding

3	cups bread cubes, firmly packed
¹/₃	cup raisins
1½	cups soymilk or rice milk
¼	cup maple syrup
1	large apple, cored and chopped

1   teaspoon vanilla
¼   teaspoon cinnamon
¼   teaspoon nutmeg
pinch salt

Combine all ingredients in a large bowl and let stand 15 minutes. Spread in a lightly oil-sprayed 9 X 9-inch baking dish and bake at 350 for 30 minutes.

Serves 6

Nutrition information per serving:
150 calories (10% from fat); 4 g protein; 30 g carbohydrate; 2 g fat; 176 mg sodium; 57 mg calcium

My Favorite Chocolate Pudding

Silken tofu makes a wonderful, creamy pudding. Look for it in your grocery store. Mori Nu is a widely distributed brand.

1   10.5-ounce package firm silken tofu
2   tablespoons cocoa
$1/_8$ teaspoon salt
$1/_3$ cup maple syrup
1   teaspoon vanilla

Place all ingredients into a blender and process until completely smooth. Spoon into small bowls and chill before serving.

Serves 4

Nutrition information per serving:
116 calories (18% from fat); 9 g protein; 15 g carbohydrate; 2 g fat; 74 mg sodium; 117 mg calcium

Indian Pudding

You'll love this delicious version of Indian Pudding.

    4   cups soymilk
    ½   cup cornmeal
    1   tablespoon molasses
    ¼   cup maple syrup
    ¼   teaspoon salt
    1   teaspoon ginger
    ½   teaspoon cinnamon

In a heavy saucepan stir cornmeal into 2 cups of soymilk and bring to a simmer. Cook over medium heat, stirring often, for 5 minutes. Stir in the molasses, maple syrup, salt, and spices. Stir in 1 additional cup of soymilk and continue cooking for 10 minutes, stirring often. Pour into a 1 ½ quart baking dish, then pour in the remaining cup of milk. Stir a few strokes to just barely mix. Bake at 350 for 30 minutes. Turn off oven. Leave the pudding in the oven with the door closed until the oven is cool. Serve warm or cold.

Serves 4

Nutrition information per serving:
147 calories (9% from fat); 4 g protein; 30 g carbohydrate; 1.5 g fat; 155 mg sodium; 82 mg calcium

Gingerbread

This gingerbread contains no added fat, yet is moist and delicious. Try serving it with hot applesauce for a real treat.

    ½   cup raisins
    ½   cup pitted dates, chopped
    1¾   cups water
    ¾   cup sugar or other sweetener

½	teaspoon salt
2	teaspoons cinnamon
1	teaspoon ginger
¾	teaspoon nutmeg
¼	teaspoon cloves
2	cups whole wheat pastry flour
1	teaspoon baking soda
1	teaspoon baking powder

Combine dried fruits, water, sugar and seasonings in a large saucepan and bring to a boil. Boil for 2 minutes, then remove from heat and cool completely.

Preheat oven to 350. Stir the flour, baking soda, and baking powder together. Add to the cooled fruit mixture and stir just to mix. Spread into a 9 X 9-inch pan which has been sprayed with a nonstick spray and bake for 30 minutes, or until a toothpick inserted into the center comes out clean.

One 9 X 9-inch cake

Nutrition information per serving:
207 calories (1% from fat); 4 g protein; 48 g carbohydrate; 0.1 g fat; 216 sodium; 52 mg calcium

Pumpkin Raisin Cookies

Children love these plump, moist cookies because they taste so good. You'll love them because they're loaded with beta-carotene and other nutrients.

3	cups whole wheat pastry flour
4	teaspoons baking powder
1	teaspoon salt
1	teaspoon baking soda
1	teaspoon cinnamon
½	teaspoon nutmeg
¾	cup sugar or other sweetener

1   15-ounce can solid-pack pumpkin
1   ripe banana, mashed
1   cup soymilk or water
1   cup raisins

Preheat oven to 350°. Mix dry ingredients together and set aside. Add the pumpkin, mashed banana, soymilk or water, and raisins. Mix until just combined.

Drop by tablespoonfuls onto a baking sheet which has been sprayed with a nonstick spray. Bake 15 minutes, until lightly browned. Remove from baking sheet with a spatula, and place on a rack to cool. Store in an airtight container.

Makes 36 3-inch cookies

Nutrition information per cookie:
75 calories (1% from fat); 1.5 g protein; 17 g carbohydrate; 0.1 g fat; 134 mg sodium; 43 mg calcium

Prune Whip

Who ever dreamed that prunes could taste so good?

1   cup prunes
1   cup water
$1/3$ cup soymilk or rice milk
3   tablespoons carob powder
2   tablespoons maple syrup

Place prunes and water in a covered saucepan and simmer until the prunes are tender, about 20 minutes. Allow to cool slightly, then transfer the prunes and any remaining liquid into a blender. Add remaining ingredients and blend until completely smooth. Spoon into small serving dishes and chill. Serves 4

Nutrition information per serving:
166 calories (2% from fat); 2 g protein; 39 g carbohydrate; 0.4 g fat; 12 mg sodium; 58 mg calcium

Baked Apples

This dessert contains no added sugar or fat, yet it is delicious and satisfying.

    4   large green apples
    5   pitted dates, chopped
    1   teaspoon cinnamon

Wash apples, then remove core to within ¼-inch of bottoms. Combine dates and cinnamon, then fill the center of each apple. Place in a baking dish filled with ¼ inch of hot water, and bake at 350° until the apples are tender when pierced with a sharp knife, 40 to 60 minutes. Serve hot or chilled.

Serves 4

Nutrition information per apple:
24 calories (3% from fat); 0.5 g protein; 29 g carbohydrate; 0.4 g fat; 0.2 mg sodium; 15 mg calcium

Poached Pears

These are delicious, and deceptively easy to prepare.

2	large ripe pears
½	cup apple juice concentrate
½	cup water
¼	teaspoon cinnamon
$1/_8$	teaspoon cloves
	non-dairy frozen dessert: Sweet Nothings, Vanilla Rice Dream or Living Lightly

Peel pears, then slice in half and remove cores. Place in a saucepan. Mix the apple juice concentrate and water with the spices, then pour over pears. Bring to a simmer over medium heat, then cover and cook until the pears are just tender when pierced with a sharp knife, about 15 minutes. Remove pears and place into individual serving dishes. Continue to simmer the juice until it is decreased by half, about 5 minutes. Pour over pears. To serve, top with a scoop of non-dairy frozen dessert.

Serves 4

Nutrition information per ½ pear:
162 calories (4% from fat); 1 g protein; 36 g carbohydrate; 1 g fat; 17 mg sodium; 17 mg calcium

Pumpkin Pie

Cornstarch is used as a thickener in place of eggs in this pie and the pie is baked in a delicious fat-free crust.

4	tablespoons cornstarch
½	cup sugar or other sweetener
½	teaspoon salt
1	teaspoon cinnamon
½	teaspoon ginger

$^1/_8$ teaspoon cloves
1½   cups cooked pumpkin
1½   cups soymilk or rice milk
1   cup Grape-Nuts cereal
¼   cup apple juice concentrate (undiluted)

Preheat oven to 350°. In a large bowl combine the cornstarch with the sugar, salt, cinnamon, ginger, and cloves. Blend in the pumpkin and milk.

In a separate bowl, mix the Grape-Nuts and apple juice concentrate. Pat into the bottom and part way up the sides of a 9-inch pie pan and bake for 7 minutes. Fill with the pumpkin mixture and bake an additional 45 minutes. Cool before cutting.

One 9-inch pie

Nutrition information per serving:
150 calories (3% from fat); 3 g protein; 33 g carbohydrate; 0.5 g fat; 186 mg sodium; 49 mg calcium

Banana Dream Pie

Ripe bananas, vanilla, and a touch of tofu make a creamy, delicious, and cholesterol-free pie.

1	cup Grape-Nuts cereal
¼	cup apple juice concentrate (undiluted)
½	cup sugar or other sweetener
5	tablespoons cornstarch
2	cups soymilk or rice milk
½	teaspoon salt
1	teaspoon vanilla
½	pound firm tofu
2	ripe bananas

Preheat oven to 350°. Mix the Grape-Nuts and apple juice concentrate, then pat into the bottom and part way up the sides of a 9-inch pie pan. Bake until edges just begin to darken, about 8 minutes. Cool.

Mix the sugar and cornstarch in a saucepan, then stir in the milk and salt. Cook over medium heat, stirring constantly, until the mixture becomes a very thick pudding. Remove from heat and stir in vanilla. Drain the tofu and blend it in a food processor until it is totally smooth, then add the pudding and blend until smooth.

Slice bananas into thin rounds over the cooled crust. Spread the tofu mixture on top. Refrigerate until completely chilled, at least two hours.

One 9-inch pie

Nutrition information per serving:
204 calories (9% from fat); 6 g protein; 42 g carbohydrate; 1.4 g fat; 255 mg sodium; 71 mg calcium

REFERENCES

1. Kendall A, Levitsky DA, Strupp BJ, Lissner L. Weight loss on a low-fat diet: consequence of the imprecision of the control of food intake in humans. Am J Clin Nutr 1991;53:1124-9.

2. Ornish D, Brown SE, Scherwitz LW, et al. Can lifestyle changes reverse coronary heart disease? Lancet 1990;336:129-133.

3. Henson LC, Poole DC, Donahoe CP, Heber D. Effects of exercise training on resting energy expenditure during caloric restriction. Am J Clin Nutr 1987;46:893-9.

4. Foster GD, et al. Controlled trial of the metabolic effects of a very-low-calorie diet: short- and long-term effects. Am J Clin Nutr 1990;51:167-72.

5. Acheson KJ, Schutz Y, Bessard T, Anantharaman K, Flatt JP, Jequier E. Glycogen storage capacity and de novo lipogenesis during massive carbohydrate overfeeding in man. Am J Clin Nutr 1988;48:240-7.

6. Horton TJ, Drougas H, Brachey A, Reed GW, Peters JC, Hill JO. Fat and carbohydrate overfeeding in humans: different effects on energy storage. Am J Clin Nutr 1995;62:19-29.

7. Danforth E, Jr., Sims EAH, Horton ES, Goldman RF. Correlation of serum triiodothyronine concentrations (T3) with dietary composition, gain in weight and thermogenesis in man. Diabetes 1975;24:406.

8. Spaulding SW, Chopra IJ, Sherwin RS, Lyall SS. Effect of caloric restriction and dietary composition on serum T3 and reverse T3 in man. J Clin Endocrinol Metab 1976;42:197-200.

9. Welle S, Lilavivathana U, Campbell RG. Increased plasma norepinephrine concentrations and metabolic rates following glucose ingestion in man. Metabolism 1980;29:806-9.

10. Mathieson RA, Walberg JL, Gwazdauskas FC, Hinkle DE, Gregg JM. The effect of varying carbohydrate content of a very-low-caloric diet on resting metabolic rate and thyroid hormones. Metabolism 1986;35:394-8.

11. Tremblay A, Lavallee N, Almeras N, Allard L, Despres JP, Bouchard C. Nutritional determinants of the increase in energy intake associated with a high-fat diet. Am J Clin Nutr 1991;53:1134-7.

12. Schutz Y, Flatt JP, Jequier E. Failure of dietary fat intake to promote fat oxidation: a factor favoring the development of obesity. Am J Clin Nutr 1989;50:307-14.

13. Tremblay A, Plourde G, Despres JP, Bouchard C. Impact of dietary fat content and fat oxidation on energy intake in humans. Am J Clin Nutr 1989;49:799-805.

14. Ascherio A, Rimm EB, Stampfer MJ, Giovannucci EL, Willett WC. Dietary intake of marine n-3 fatty acids, fish intake, and the risk of coronary disease among men. N Engl J Med 1995;332:977-82.

15. de Castro JM, Orozco S. Moderate alcohol intake and spontaneous eating patterns of humans: evidence of unregulated supplementation. Am J Clin Nutr 1990;52:246-53.

16. Suter PM, Schutz Y, Jequier E. The effect of ethanol on fat storage in healthy subjects. New Engl J Med 1992;326:983-7.

17. Stunkard AJ, Harris JR, Pedersen NL, McClearn GE. The body-mass index of twins who have been reared apart. N Engl J Med 1990;322:1483-7.

18. Liebowitz MR, Klein DF. Hysteroid dysphoria. Psych Clin N Am 1979;2:555-75.

19. Michener W, Rozin P. Pharmacological versus sensory factors in the satiation of chocolate craving. Physiol Behav 1994;56:419-22.

20. Weil A. Natural Health, Natural Medicine, Houghton Mifflin, Boston, 1990, p. 145.

21. Michell GF, Mebane AH, Billings CK. Effect of bupropion on chocolate craving. Am J Psychiatry 1989;146:119-20.

22. Tomelleri R, Grunewald KK. Menstrual cycle and food cravings in young college women. J Am Dietetic Asso 1987;87:311-5.

23. Abraham GE, Lubran MM. Serum and red cell magnesium levels in patients with premenstrual tension. Am J Clin Nutr 1981;34:2364-6.

24. American Dietetic Association. Position of the American Dietetic Association on vegetarian diets. J Am Dietetic Asso 1993;93:1317-19.

25. Abelow BJ, Holford TR, Insogna KL. Cross-cultural association between dietary animal protein and hip fracture: a hypothesis. Calcif Tissue Int 1992;50:14-18.

26. Remer T, Manz F. Estimation of the renal net acid excretion by adults consuming diets containing variable amounts of protein. Am J Clin Nutr 1994;59:1356-61.

27. Nordin BEC, Need AG, Morris HA, Horowitz M. The nature and significance of the relationship between urinary sodium and urinary calcium in women. J Nutr 1993;123:1615-1622.

28. Massey LK, Whiting SJ. Caffeine, urinary calcium, calcium metabolism and bone. J Nutr 1993;123:1611-4.

29. Hopper JL, Seeman E. The bone density of female twins discordant for tobacco use. N Engl J Med 1994;330:387-92.

30. Broadus AE. Mineral metabolism. In: Felig P, Baxter JD, Broadus AE, Frohman LA. Endocrinology and metabolism. McGraw-Hill, New York, 1981.

31. Riggs BL, Wahner HW, Melton J, Richelson LS, Judd HL, O'Fallon M. Dietary calcium intake and rates on bone loss in women. J Clin Invest 1987;80:979-82.

32. Dawson-Hughes B, Jacques P, Shipp C. Dietary calcium intake and bone loss from the spine in healthy postmenopausal women. Am J Clin Nutr 1987;46:685-7.

33. Dawson-Hughes B. Calcium supplementation and bone loss: a review of controlled clinical trials. Am J Clin Nutr 1991;54:274S-80S.

34. Mazess RB, Barden HS. Bone density in premenopausal women: effects of age, dietary intake, physical activity, smoking, and birth-control pills. Am J Clin Nutr 1991;53:132-42.

35. Heaney RP, Weaver CM. Calcium absorption from kale. Am J Clin Nutr 1990;51:656-7.

36. Nicar MJ, Pak CYC. Calcium bioavailability from calcium carbonate and calcium citrate. J Clin Endocrinol Metab 1985;61:391-3.

37. Kissileff HR, Pi-Sunyer FX, Segal K, Meltzer S, Foelsch PA. Acute effects of exercise on food intake in obese and nonobese women. Am J Clin Nutr 1990;52:240-5.

INDEX